Pearls for Nursing Practice

Pearls for nursing practice:

a choice collection of tips, hints, timesavers, improvisations and bright ideas that make nursing easier and patients happier

Arlene Odom Nichols, R.N., B.S.N., M.S.N.
Assistant Professor
College of Nursing
The J. Hillis Miller Health Center
University of Florida, Gainesville, Florida

Joy Day, R.N., B.S.N.
Supervisor, Surgical Specialty
Shands Teaching Hospital
Gainesville, Florida

Illustrations by Connie Ardiff Barnhill, R.N.

Photographs by Chris Zimmerman

J. B. Lippincott Company
Philadelphia   New York   Toronto

Paperbound: ISBN 0-397-54251-8
Hardbound: ISBN 0-397-54338-7

Library of Congress Catalog Card Number 79-15387

Printed in the United States of America

2 4 6 8 9 7 5 3 1

Library of Congress Cataloging in Publication Data

Nichols, Arlene Odom.
    Pearls for nursing practice.

    Bibliography: p.
    1. Nursing—Handbooks, manuals, etc. I. Day, Joy,
joint author. II. Title.
RT51.N58   610.73   79-15387
Paperbound: ISBN 0-397-54251-8
Hardbound: ISBN 0-397-54338-7

Contents

Unit II Pearls for Special Problems 101

Unit III Pearls for Nursing Management 177

Foreword

Professional nurses in the business of delivering nursing care to patients, directly or indirectly, represent a too often untapped and unshared reservoir of information to accomplish patient care objectives. This information includes the "pearls" presented in this book—tips and techniques which can facilitate the delivery of individualized care with the greatest efficiency, ease and benefit to patient and nurse.

The presentation of pearls includes not only what to do but also some of the "why" or rationale for a particular approach. This is an important positive aspect of this book, as it removes some of the mystique which may surround actions of a confident practicing nurse being observed by a student or a new graduate. This book also represents excellent collaborative efforts between professional nurses in a service setting and professional nurses in an educational setting. The results can benefit nursing students, new graduates, and experienced practicing professionals.

Beverly Keene, R.N., M.N., Director of Nursing Services,
Shands Teaching Hospital, Gainesville, Florida

Like their namesake, the pearls included in this volume represent responses to a problem. They should be valued as gems for they reflect the expertise of nurses in accomplishing nursing goals through effective and often creative means.

It is through the talents of the practitioner that we improve practice. It is through the medium of books that we share those improvements with our colleagues. The contributors are to be commended for their participation in a reference devoted to the practical aspects of nursing.

Blanche Urey, R.N., Ed.D.
Dean and Professor
University of Florida
College of Nursing

Preface

As we near the completion of this book, a fair question to ask would be, "How did we ever think we might be able to write a book?" Looking back over what we have done, I'm amazed at how easy we thought it would be. It all happened one day when Arlene, with her students said to Joy, with her staff, about a particularly unique way of doing something, "We ought to write that down, in fact, we ought to write a book of things like that." Joy said, "Hey, you're right." So we called up the fine Nursing Editor at the J. B. Lippincott Publishing Company. He said, "That's a good idea." and we wrote a book. The staff at the hospital and the students and instructors at the College of Nursing poured in their hints, their tips, their pearls, and we started to work.

So, to answer the question, "Who are we to write a book?" we are nobody special except two nurses who had a good idea and followed through on it; but the tip-givers, the body of people of whom we are a part, are very special indeed. They are a group of people who have quietly gone about the business of caring for sick people and noticing little tricks that seemed to make things work better. The wealth of their knowledge is barely tapped—and it is considerable. What we have tried to do is to share with you, in an organized fashion, a small portion of the ideas, the pearls that we found.

Here is a sketch of what is enclosed between these covers:

There are a few old, old tips, like the easiest way to put on a pillowcase and the best way to give a back-rub, that stand in danger of being lost to generations of new nurses who may not be in a position to hear (or inclined to listen) to their elders. These are a part of nursing tradition, but we were surprised at the number of people who had forgotten or had never heard of them. We decided to compile these ideas in our book. We do so with a very respectful salute to those who told us.

There are some tips so new that they are just barely considered within the realm of nursing practice—like "Cannulating High Pressure Arteriovenous Fistulae"—provided for us by nurses who are breaking new ground for the profession by pioneering in expanded roles. To them also we tip our caps.

There are tips from specialists who have learned by practice, by organizing with their fellow specialists, by becoming absorbed in their particular fields, to be very, very good at what they do. We are amazed at the growth that has occurred in specialties that were formerly not considered specialties at all. So, to the specialists, our thanks and our admiration.

And tips from generalists, who prefer to think of themselves as "Renaissance People," bringing as much knowledge of as many fields as they can to each of their patients. One can almost never successfully argue with these people, so rich and varied is their experience.

We cannot forget the allied health professions. Several in particular—the dietary department, physical therapy department, and speech and hearing section—gave us some valuable pearls. They were in fact eager to share with us the things regarding patient care that they had learned. Perhaps interdisciplinary communication such as this needs to occur on a more routine basis.

The ideas in this book all came from the health care people at the Shands Teaching Hospital and Clinics and the J. Hillis Miller Health Center at the University of Florida. We are sure that they are just a few of the pearls in the total scope of nursing practice. Perhaps you have some of your own that are as good, or even better. If you would like to, feel free to write to us about them.

Just a quick reminder: no book of pearls, helpful hints, etc. can function as a substitute for sound nursing judgment. As always the professional nurse must assess the patient's needs and apply the appropriate nursing intervention based on his analysis of the individual situation with which he is confronted. Seen in this light, the pearls we have presented are the shared knowledge of health professionals who have faced common "problem" situations and used innovative solutions.

Acknowledgments

Our special thanks go to:

Mr. David T. Miller, Managing Editor, Nursing Department, J. B. Lippincott Company, who we found to be a real gem. This remarkable man has the keen ability of fostering motivation and perseverence in the writers through his genuinely shared enthusiasm, wit and guidance.

We are greatly indebted to Collette Joy Ralston for her typing and assistance in the preparation of this manuscript.

And for those valuable pearls we acknowledge Joyce Stechmiller, for her major contribution to the sharing of Pearls in the Health Education chapter, and the following contributors, all from the J. Hillis Miller Health Center, University of Florida:

Gloria Jean Allen, R.N., Cardiovascular Nursing (VA)

Susan Arline, RN.., Surgical Specialties

Winkie Atkinson, R.N., Emergency Room

V. Bailey, L.P.N., Surgical Nursing (VA)

Connie Barnhill, R.N., General Surgery

Dorothy Barrus, R.N., Pediatrics, 7th Floor

Paul Beattie, R.P.T., Physical Therapy

Jodi Benedette, R.N., MICU/CCU

Carroll Bennett, Professor, College of Dentistry

Bruce Boswell, R.N., Surgical Intensive Care Unit

Scott Brannon, Manager, Health Center Stores

Robert Cade, M.D., College of Medicine

Veronica Carr, R.N., Staff Development

Hester Cecil, Assistant Manager, CSR

Gloria Chiras, R.N., Assistant Professor, College of Nursing

Pat Clunn, R.N., Assistant Professor Psych/Mental Health, College of Nursing

Myrna Courage, R.N., Visiting Assistant Professor, College of Nursing Psych/Mental Health

Robin Crawford, S.N., College of Nursing

Marsha Cummings, R.D., Nutritional Services

Frances Daniels, N.A., Surgical Specialties

Harriet Daniels, R.N., Assistant Director, Nursing

Marti Davies, R.N., Pediatrics

George A. Dell, M.D., Pediatrician

Shirley (Pat) Dixon, R.N., Oncological Clinician

Paul Doering, M.S.R., Phar., College of Pharmacy

Hugh Dole, R.T., Respiratory Therapy

Margaret Duerson, R.N., Department of Surgery

Cathy Edelstein, R.N., General Surgery
Myra Eden, R.N., Supervisor, NICU
Cindy Emerman, S.N., College of Nursing
Annette Frauman, R.N., Adult Nursing
    Practitioner, Assistant Professor,
    College of Nursing
Gail Gatch, R.N., Operating Room
Sheila Gerwirtz, R.N., College of Nursing
Kathie Gilbert, L.P.N., Postanesthesia
    Recovery Room
Cyrena Gilman, R.N., Supervisor, Pediatrics
    Dialysis
Karolyn Godbey, R.N., Assistant Professor,
    Psych/Mental Health, College of
    Nursing
Karen Mack Goff, R.N., General Surgery
George Golay, R.T.N., Pediatrics
Janice Goodwin, R.P.T., Physical Therapy
Peggy Guin, R.N., Surgical Specialties
Debra Hague, S.N., College of Nursing
Melanie Halfaker, R.N., Burn Unit
June Alice Halls, L.P.N., PICU
Marta Hammond, S.N., College of Nursing
Carol Hayes, R.N., Associate Professor,
    College of Nursing
Louise Hill, L.P.N., Surgical Nursing (VA)
Essie Hodges, Unit Manager, General
    Surgery
Janice Holmes, R.N., Surgical Nursing (VA)
Thelma Holmes, R.P.T., Physical Therapy
Edna Hotton, N.A., Surgical Specialties
Ann Hudson, R.N. (Enterostomal Therapist),
    Staff Development
Mary Jackson, R.N., MICU
Linda Jenkins, L.P.N., MICU
Rae Ann Kaylor, R.N., Surgical Specialties
Lois Knowles, R.N., Professor, Geriatric
    Nursing, College of Nursing
Jeffery Lange, S.N., College of Nursing
Marsha Lindenbaum, R.N., Surgical
    Specialties
Meg Little, R.N., Supervisor, Burn Unit
Virginia Little, R.N., Postanesthesia
    Recovery Room
Mary Lynn, R.N., Doctoral
    Candidate/Graduate Teaching
    Assistant, College of Nursing
Denise Maifield, R.N., NICU

Jan McCurry, R.N., General Surgery
Regina McDonnell, R.N., SICU Supervisor
Beverly Miller, R.P.T., Physical Therapy
Geraldine Miller, R.N., Cardiovascular
    Nursing (VA)
Virginia Myers, Patient Services
    Representative
Jim North, R.N., Psychiatric Nursing
Mimi Odom, R.N., Graduate Student,
    Psychiatric Nursing, College
    of Nursing
Jennie Van Orden, R.N., Surgical Specialties
Louise E. Okken, R.N., Postanesthesia
    Recovery Room
Mary Helen Owen, R.D., Nutritional
    Services
Virgie Pafford, R.N., Associate Professor,
    Community Health
Margaret Page, R.N., Emergency Room
Ellen Patterson, R.N., Nursing Practitioner
    (MIH), College of Nursing
Ruby Puckett, R.D. Director, Nutritional
    Services
Rhoda Reed, R.N., Supervisor, Pediatrics
Catherine Reilly, R.N., Instructor, MIH,
    College of Nursing
Jean Ritter, R.N., Postanesthesia Recovery
    Room
Pearlie Roberts, N.A., Surgical Specialties
June Ronga, R.N., Supervisor
Lari Ruther, L.P.N., SICU
Cindy Sager, S.N., College of Nursing
Gerrie Scully, R.N., Instructor, Medical-
    Surgical Nursing, College of Nursing
Charlotte Sharp, R.N., SICU (Inservice)
Joan Shinkus, R.N., Supervisor, SICU
Natalie Small, Pediatric Health Educator
Joy Smith, Manager, CSR
Sue Sperling, R.P.T., Director, Physical
    Therapy
Joyce Stechmiller, R.N., Assistant Professor,
    College of Nursing
Willie Stevens, N.A., Surgical (VA)
Carol Stewart, R.N., SICU
Nancy Sypert, R.N., Assistant Professor
    (Medical-Surgical), College of Nursing
Dorothy Thomas, R.N., Cardiovascular
    Nursing (VA)

Acknowledgments xv

Mary Nell Thomas, R.N., Surgical
   Specialties
Vickie Thomas, R.N., Postanesthesia
   Recovery Room
Leah Tirabassi, R.N., Emergency Room
Melinda Tocci, R.N., MICU
Helen Unser, R.D., Nutritional Services
Cindy Vaughn, R.N., Postanesthesia
   Recovery Room

Karen Verhoeve, S.N., College of Nursing
Jim Wagner, Chaplain Director,
   Pastoral Care
Peggy Wilson, R.N., Assistant Professor
   (Pediatric Nursing), College
   of Nursing
Diana Wren, R.N., Labor/Delivery (MIH)
Gladys Wyman, R.N., Assistant Director,
   Nursing Service

Participants in the photographic sessions:
Heather Barbour, R.N., MICU/CCU
Elouise Foster, N.A., Surgical Specialties
Melanie Halfaker, R.N., Burn Unit
Sandra Katrina, R.N., Instructor, Pediatrics,
   College of Nursing
Sandra B. Lavoie, R.P.T., Physical Therapy
Meg Little, R.N., Supervisor, Burn Unit
Rae Maren, R.N., Medical Supervisor
Mary Morris, Administrative Secretary
Anne Neven, Clerk, Burn Unit

Jean Ritter, R.N., Postanesthesia Recovery
   Room
Clem Robillard, R.N., Surgical Specialties
Anita T. Salzberg, R.P.T., Physical
   Therapy
Jerry Sercey, N.A., Surgical Specialties
Vickie Thomas, R.N., Postanesthesia
   Recovery Room
Leah Wacksman, R.N., Ophthalmology
   Supervisor

Pearls for Nursing Practice

Pearls for
basic
needs

Unit I

Mobility

Chapter one

The *freedom of movement* is often viewed as congruent with life itself. We find evidence of this in the glowing expression of joy in the expectant mother as she experiences first fetal movements; the parental delight over the child's first step; the teenager's newest dance contortion to the latest hit record; and the well-trod paths of the joggers.

The patient's mobility is dependent on the functioning of an intact neuromusculoskeletal system and his ability to control his movements without injury. Consequently, movement (mobility) is an essential part of holistic man.

Immobility is the loss of this freedom of movement. Such loss or alteration may be the result of:

1. Stressors (such as illness) which limit the patient's ability to control his mobility.
2. Restrictions ordered to conserve energy and promote restoration.
3. Trauma or disease to the neuromusculoskeletal system itself.

As nurses, we are often dealing with patients who are in a state of altered mobility. We find ourselves at the two extremes: either encouraging mobility in the patient or actually restricting his mobility.

This chapter shares pearls which you will find helpful as you care for your patients with altered mobility.

Use the pearls as you find them helpful in attaining the following goals of care for your individual patient:

1. Promoting an optimum level of activity
2. Application of good body mechanics as care is given
3. Prevention of complications
4. Minimizing problems of altered mobility

AMBULATION
Pearl (1) Who's Walking Whom?

Many patients who lack strength or stability to walk alone find assistance from another person very supportive. Despite good intentions, we too often see the patient being assisted incorrectly (Figure 1-1).

A correct, safe and more effective way of assisting the patient is shown in Figure 1-2.

What points should be emphasized when assisting with ambulation?

1. The patient is positioned near a wall or other supportive structure. (Should he become weak, he can be supported against this wall.)
2. The patient places the weight of one hand in the nurse's hand. (It helps to tell the patient this at the outset.) This provides a focal point which encourages balance, as it lowers the center of gravity and allows for greater support and control to turn around or if the patient tires suddenly.
3. The nurse and the patient step simultaneously on opposite feet. This will allow the nurse to support the patient against the wall, should it become necessary, by locking his knee with her leg (Figure 1-3).
4. When the arms are around the waist rather than over the shoulders or about the neck (which encourages slouching and decreases control of the situation), you will find the patient tires less quickly, because his good posture permits better oxygenation from adequate chest expansion.

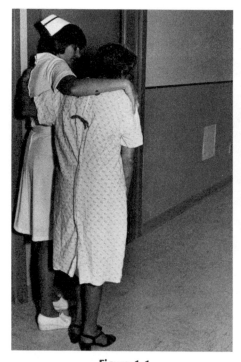

Figure 1-1

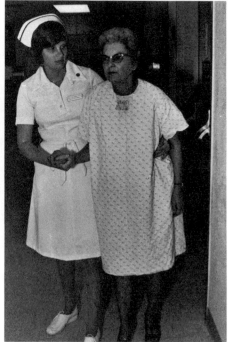

Figure 1-2

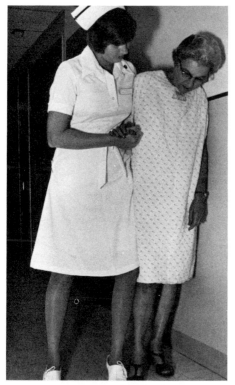 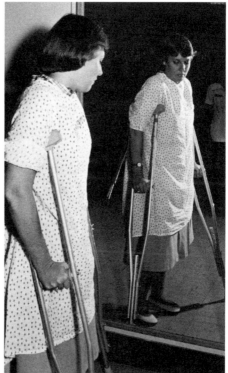

Figure 1-3   Figure 1-4

Pearl (2) That Mirror-Image

A full-length stationary or portable mirror serves as a valuable aid in helping the patient maintain good posture and in providing him feedback about his appearance (Figure 1-4). Some situations in which we have found this very useful include:
1. The postoperative patient with an abdominal incision who is trying to walk erect.
2. The woman who has had a mastectomy and is performing arm exercises and practicing posture.
3. The patient who is crutch-walking.
4. The child with scoliosis who is performing pelvic-tilt exercises.
5. The patient with a colostomy, who is learning self-care. This also permits him to view himself fully dressed for any telltale signs of the stomal devices. It fosters a better self-image and encourages mobility—getting out of the room and "meeting the world."

As you can see, there are numerous situations in which you will find such a mirror useful.

Pearl (3) 3 S's for Ambulating (Safety, Support, *Shoes*)

Avoid ambulating the patient in his bare feet. Have him wear his shoes. Shoes help to prevent injury and provide support.

Pearl (4) Tape the Soles for Friction

Some hospitals provide inexpensive disposable shoes. When no shoes are available and ambulation should be practiced, place a piece of adhesive tape on the soles of patients' feet. This provides some friction and prevents slipping (Figure 1-5).

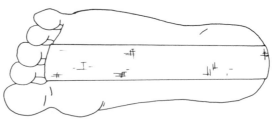

Figure 1-5

Pearl (5) Foot Drop—A Deterrent to Ambulating

For the patients who have foot drop (from hemiparesis, etc.) easier ambulation with less potential for injury to the affected foot will result if you will wrap an ace bandage around the forefoot and secure the bandage so that the foot is lifted slightly upward and does not drag. It is necessary to check the dressing to prevent ischemia from occurring because of the dressing's tightness.

Pearl (6) Plotting the Route

To encourage motivation in the early school-age child to increase his level of mobility, a map of the route to be traveled, with destination and landmarks, is drawn and planned with the youngster. He then colors that portion he travels at selected times (usually daily), using a different color for each time. This helps him become more aware of his progress. It is posted at his bedside for him to share with his parents and others. Such a map can be altered to meet the developmental level and physical capabilities of the child.

Pearl (7) Ambulating with the Arm Elevated

Occasionally you find a patient who needs to ambulate and whose arm must remain elevated for various reasons. Both goals can be accomplished by suspending the patient's arm from a portable IV pole with stockinette.

Pearl (8) First Ambulation—Promote Venous Return

Wrap an ace bandage about the legs or use thromboembolic deterrent (TED) stockings on the patient who is to ambulate for the first time after being on bedrest. This promotes venous return.

BEDREST
Pearl (9) Turning Made Easier

You will find that turning the helpless patient is more easily accomplished if pressure is applied simultaneously on the lateral portion of the flexed knee and posteriorly on the upper extremity (Figure 1-6). (Of course, you are remembering to use your principles of good body mechanics at all times as you position your patients.)

Pearl (10) The Pillow Takes a Position Change

Before you begin to turn the patient on his side when making the bed or repositioning the patient, change the placement of the pillow. This provides a continuous support to the head and neck (Figure 1-6). The pillow should be placed so that one end is under the patient's head and the bulk of the pillow is extended on the side to which the patient is to be turned.

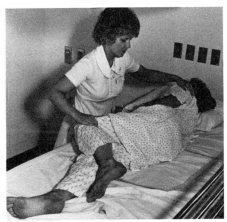

Figure 1-6

Pearl (11) Tucking the Pillow Support

The following steps describe how to place a pillow against the patient's back as a support in keeping him in a lateral position.

1. Place a pillow lengthwise so that each end helps in supporting joints and bones as it supports the back. The upper edge should be at the lower scapular area (right below arm pits) and the lower edge should reach the iliac crest. (Occasionally two pillows will be required for patients with long torsos.)

2. Push the side of the pillow nearest the patient downward, tucking the edge snugly against his back and the bottom sheet.

3. Then begin to roll the pillow (from the side nearer to you) under while pushing against it toward the patient. This helps to prevent the pillow slipping and unrolling and provides comfortable back support.

Pearl (12) The Lift Sheet and Sheepskin

Fold a sheet lengthwise and place it under the patient's hips to aid in moving him in bed (a draw sheet may be used without being folded). Keep the edges fan-folded on each side of the bed.

When beginning to lift the patient to move him toward the head of the bed, roll the edges of the sheet toward the patient or toward the center of the bed. Using good body mechanics, rock to and fro on each count (count aloud) and move the patient using the lift sheet on the count of *three*.

Sheepskin can be used in an effort to prevent decubiti and as a lift sheet. When sheepskins are used, their effectiveness is lost if they are covered with sheets, Chux, etc.

Pearl (13) Up in Bed

Since use of a Gatch bed can lead to circulatory stasis, this practice is discouraged. Alternatives include:
1. Frequent repositioning of the patient
2. Use of a footboard
3. Use of improvised footboards such as:
    a. placement of the headboard proximal to the footboard of the bed with a pillow between the two.
    b. rolling a bath blanket across the foot of the bed and securing it so that the patient's feet can rest against it.

Pearl (14) Prone Positioning for Amputee

To prevent contractures and to promote hyperextension, the patient who has a lower extremity amputation must be on his abdomen at intervals, when at all possible.

In addition, the patient should avoid keeping the stump in a flexed position. To prevent flexion contractures, when the patient is sitting, *discourage* the placement of any pad, pillow, etc. under the stump which elevates it.

Pearl (15) Directions for Turning

To save valuable time and provide a reasonable position-change schedule for your patient, keep a position chart taped to the head of the bed. The chart indicates the time for turning as well as illustrates the various positions to be used for individual patients. You will find this is helpful for any patient who requires frequent turning in bed.

The positions can be numbered on the chart and recorded after each position change on the flow sheet at the bedside.

Pearl (16) Chaise Longue Position for Patients with Total Hip Replacement

To prevent displacement of the ball and socket (the prosthesis in the acetabulum) in the patient who is recuperating following a total hip replacement, ensure that the patient avoids sitting in a Fowler's (i.e., a straight chair) type position but rather *sits in a chaise longue position*. When a chaise longue is not available, improvise by having the patient use an overstuffed chair which is not upright and place pillows so that his feet are up on a stool or other chair. An *adjustable* back wheelchair (like the old wooden wheel chairs) can be altered to provide such a position when the patient's feet are placed on the bed, which is completely lowered, or on a stool.

USING CRUTCHES
Pearl (17) Stepping Off with Crutches

Until your patient has had enough practice using his new crutches, give him assistance to prevent falls and yet get the feel of balancing on his own with them (Figure 1-7).

1. Walk behind the patient. In this way you can grab him around the waist if he begins to fall.

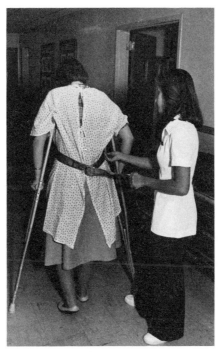

Figure 1-7

2. Use a rope belt (made from rope, Kerlix, or a drawsheet, etc.) to wrap around the patient's waist. (A patient's own belt can be used without the need for "looping" for the same purpose.)

Following are essentials for safe crutch walking.

Pearl (18) Safe Walkway

The area should be cleared of gadgets that may cause the patient to trip and fall (e.g., electrical cords, footstools, throw rugs, etc.) when learning to maneuver with his crutches.

Pearl (19) No Instructions—No Crutches

Never give a patient a pair of crutches without proper instructions and fitting. The weight of the body should be on the hands—*not* at the elbow or the axilla.

Remove the padding from the shoulder piece of the crutch to discourage weight bearing at that point. Such incorrect use of crutches can lead to permanent nerve damage at the axilla.

Pearl (20) Shifting Weight

Have the patient practice shifting weight side to side with the use of crutches before actually walking.

Pearl (21) Observing Crutch Stance

Observe the patient using crutches:

1. If the patient's shoulders are elevated, the crutches are too long (Figure 1-8).
2. If the patient appears hunched the crutches are probably too short (Figure 1-9).
3. Teach the patient crutch walking before a *full length mirror* (Figure 1-10).

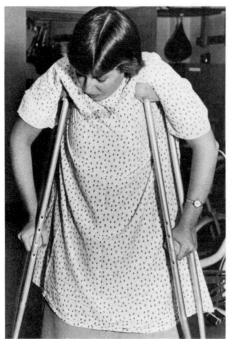
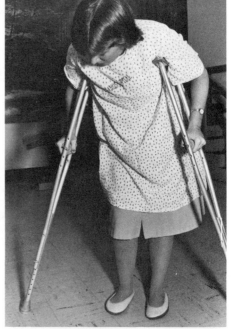
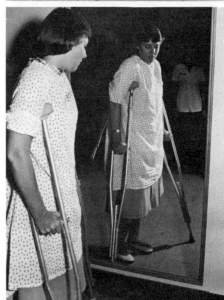

Figure 1-8 (top left)
Figure 1-9 (top right)
Figure 1-10 (bottom)

Pearl (22) Fitting the Crutches

When available, the physical therapist should fit the patient for crutches and teach him to use them. On many occasions the nurse is in situations in which she must assume this responsibility. This is particularly true in instances where crutches will be needed for only short-term use (e.g., when the young teenage athlete sprains an ankle and is treated at the local clinic or emergency room).

There are different methods used for measuring the patient for crutches. When possible, have the patient stand. Measure from the axilla to a point about six inches out from the side of the heel. Provide a two-inch gap between the axilla and the shoulder piece. The hand grip should be positioned so there is a 15 to 30 degree flexion of the elbows when standing. Flexion decreases (but still within the 15 to 30 degree range) with increased weight bearing. The crutch tips should be positioned three to four inches out from each side of the patient and about three to four inches in front of him.

TRANSFERRING SAFELY
Pearl (23) Repositioning from a Slide in the Chair

Note in Figures 1-11 and 1-12 a maneuver which prevents strain and trauma to the patient or yourself, as you reposition him in his chair. The essential steps include:

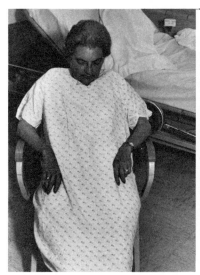
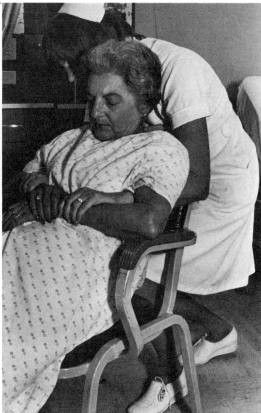

Figure 1-11 (top)
Figure 1-12 (right)

1. The nurse stands behind the patient's chair.
2. She slips her arms around the patient, reaching under his arms.
3. She grasps his forearms and folds them upon each other.
4. Then the nurse flexes her knees and lifts the patient backward and upward in the chair.

   This saves the nurse's back and the patient's skin.

Pearl (24) The Rubber Mat

The use of a nonskid rubber mat under the patient's feet helps to prevent sliding in the chair.

Pearl (25) A Sheet to Save a Slide

Another way to keep the patient from sliding in the chair is to fold a sheet, on the bias, and place it across his chest and under his arms. Then tie the ends of the sheet to the top of the back of the chair. The placement of the sheet can be altered when necessary, to extend around the patient's waist instead of his chest (Figure 1-13).

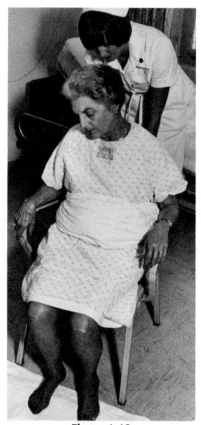

Figure 1-13

Pearl (26) Transfer of the Amputee from Bed to Chair

Make the transfer of the patient with bilateral amputation of the lower extremities safer and simpler for the patient and the nurse by turning the wheelchair to face the bed and filling the gap between the bed and chair with a pillow. Adjust the bed's height as needed and lock the wheelchair. The patient backs into the wheelchair while lifting himself with his hands on the arms of the chair (Figure 1-14).

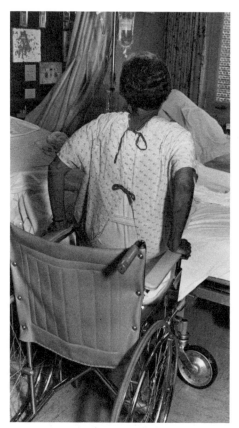

Figure 1-14

Pearl (27) Instruct—Push with Feet

When assisting the weak patient in getting out of the chair, instruct him to *push* with his feet. Many times the patient assumes you will lift him when he may be quite able to assist in providing the momentum needed to stand when instructed to do so.

Pearl (28) Transfer Toward "Good" Side

Move the patient toward his strong side when transferring. Also *watch out* for and provide support for the weakened extremities. This tip is particularly useful in the care of the patient with hemiparesis or hemiplegia, such as the stroke patient.

TRANSFERRING IN AN EMERGENCY
Pearl (29) A Safe Move from the Back Seat

When a patient must be transferred from the back seat of a car to the emergency room (ER) by stretcher, a minimum of two people is required.

Both enter the car from doors on opposite sides of the car, then they slide the patient out in a *straight* line, using a two-man or three-man lift.

Pearl (30) Getting the Patient *Off* the Floor

When you find the patient lying on the floor and you (alone) must get him up into a chair or on a bed, place the chair on the floor (Figure 1-15). Carefully pull the patient into the chair. Then secure the patient in the chair with a restraint (Figure 1-16). Set the chair upright (Figure 1-17). This is easier and safer for the patient and you than attempting to transfer the patient alone from the floor to the bed or chair.

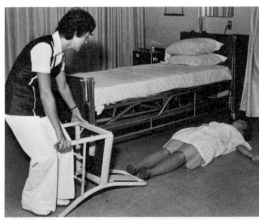

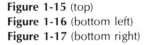

Figure 1-15 (top)
Figure 1-16 (bottom left)
Figure 1-17 (bottom right)

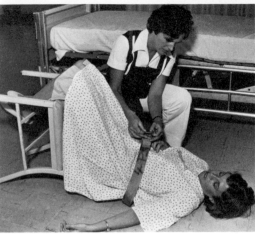

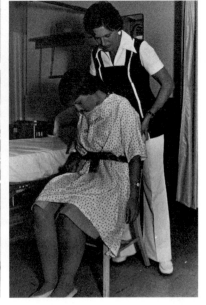

INNOVATIONS WITH ASSISTIVE DEVICES
Pearl (31) Chair Substitute for Parallel Bars

When a patient needs parallel bars for ambulating and none are available, line chairs side by side to serve as a substitute (Figure 1-18).

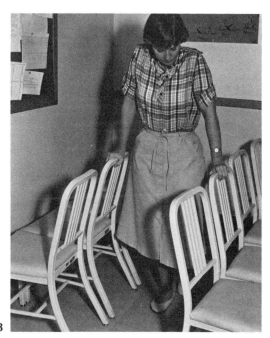

Figure 1-18

Pearl (32) Children, Broomsticks, Chairs

For children who need the use of parallel bars for ambulating, place broomsticks between chairs when no bars are available (Figure 1-19).

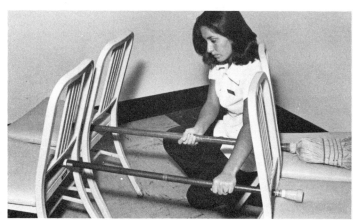

Figure 1-19

Pearl (33) Reversed Walker Becomes a Support Bar

Reverse the walker, place it over the commode and the weak patient has a readily accessible device to help lower and lift himself on and off the commode (Figure 1-20).

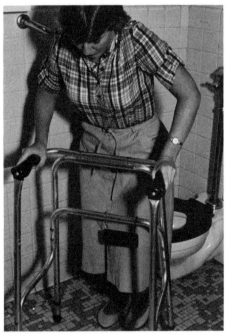

Figure 1-20

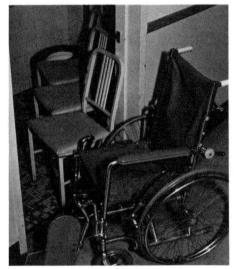

Figure 1-21

Pearl (34) The Slide in a Chair Train

When the wheelchair will not fit through a narrow bathroom doorway, place chairs side by side. The patient can transfer from chair to chair to the commode (Figure 1-21).

Pearl (35) The Old Red Wagon Ain't What It Used to Be

Mobilizing an ill child can be challenging. How about a wagon ride? The pediatric unit uses large wagons, cushioned with pillows, with IV poles attached. The sides are high enough to keep the child from falling out. It is more familiar and less threatening than a wheelchair, and a whole lot more fun than a stretcher. Parents and nurses can easily pull the patient around the unit, or take him to the playroom to visit other patients (Figure 1-22).

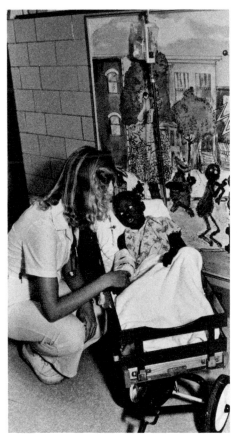

Figure 1-22

EXERCISE
Pearl (36) Overexercising Can Be Harmful

More and more the geriatric patient is becoming cognizant of good health practices. While "jogging" and other physical exercise have become an increasing American pastime, the patient must be taught the hazards of overexercising and a sensible daily exercise program to meet his individual needs.

Pearl (37) Squeezing the Rubber Ball

Using a *soft* rubber ball for hand exercise is satisfactory *if* the patient has *active* motion in the hand (e.g., patient with fractures of lower extremities who will need to crutch walk). For those patients who *do not* have active hand motion (e.g., the stroke patient with hemiparesis, etc.), a large syringe container or other hard object is preferred. This squeezing of the *soft* rubber ball in patients *without* active hand motion is to be *discouraged* as it increases the spasticity and the possibility of contractures.

Pearl (38) Strengthening the Triceps

Many patients need exercise to strengthen those triceps muscles used for crutch walking. If trapeze bars are eliminated, the in-bed patient will use his triceps rather than the biceps to raise himself up in bed and move about the bed. By using his hands to push himself from a dorsal to sitting position, and by lifting his buttocks as he shifts from side to side in the bed, he will be exercising the triceps.

CAST CARE
Pearl (39) Petaling the Cast

Once dry, the cast edges should be covered either with stockinette or by "petaling." This prevents skin abrasions from the rough edges of the cast or from the plaster chips.

To make petals the easy way (and, by the way, an ample supply of these could be made in advance):
1. Cut the desired length of three-inch adhesive tape.
2. Place the adhesive strip onto a sheet of plastic or waxed paper.
3. Mark off two-inch strips on the tape.
4. Round edges (Figure 1-23, left).
5. Cut strips and apply over the edges of the cast, slightly overlapping each petal (Figure 1-23, right).

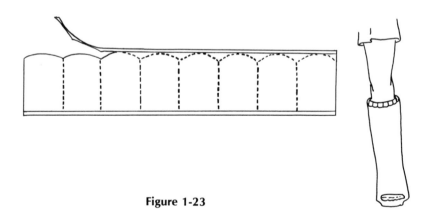

Figure 1-23

Pearl (40) Scratching Safely

Prior to cast application in the operating room, suggest to the physician that he include a strip of flannel which will extend four to six inches beyond the proximal and distal ends of the cast.

This will discourage the patient from placing objects underneath the cast to scratch. He can now use the soft "scratch flannel" by pulling slightly back and forth.

Pearl (41) Fanning the Itch

A portable hair blower turned to *cool setting only* can force air under the edges of cast to aid in eliminating itching. This also serves to deter the patient from placing gadgets which could be quite harmful underneath the cast.

RESTRAINTS

Alteration in mobility may be a deliberate part of restrictions which are ordered to conserve patient energy, prevent injury and promote restorations. One of the difficult situations which the nurse must deal with is that occasion when the use of restraints become necessary for the patient's well-being. The following ten pearls are examples of how safe restraints can be made and applied.

Pearl (42) Making a Restraint

1. Take "A" and "B" and place them side by side.
2. Slip over the extremity (Figure 1-24).
3. Pull ends taut, safely.
4. Tie the ends to an armboard or bed (never to side rails).

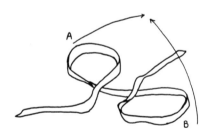

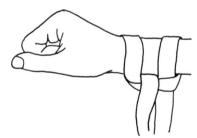

Figure 1-24

Pearl (43) The Restraint Which Never Pulls Too Tightly

This restraint can be enlarged or tightened by pulling one end at a time. Pulling both ends, simultaneously, does not alter the restraint. Steps:

1. Drape gauze strip (Kerlix) over one hand with the longer portion falling posteriorly over the hand (Figure 1-25).
2. With the other hand grasp the longer portion of the Kerlix.
3. Hands should be at the same level (Figure 1-26).
4. Slip one hand with Kerlix through the loop of Kerlix in the other hand (Figure 1-27).

Now you are ready to slide the restraint over the extremity and alter the restraint to the size needed to fit correctly.

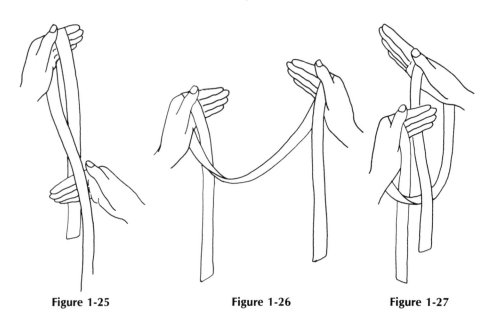

Figure 1-25   Figure 1-26   Figure 1-27

Pearl (44) Using the Posey Restraint

When you need to restrain a child, use a Posey tie-back or a safety vest when at all possible. This is better tolerated by the child than placing all four extremities in restraints. (This product is available from J.T. Posey Company.)

Pearl (45) A Quick Soft Restraint

Here is a soft restraint that can be made quickly out of material which is readily available on most nursing units.

Materials needed for one restraint: one abdominal dressing (ABD) pad; one Kling or Kerlix roll; wide (three-inch) adhesive tape.

1. Fold the ABD pad in half lengthwise.
2. Unroll the Kling or Kerlix bandage and place it perpendicular to the patient's arm or leg at the wrist or ankle, approximately centered.
3. Wrap the ABD pad snugly around the wrist or ankle, covering with the

Kling or Kerlix. If the patient's wrist or ankle is so large that the ABD pad will not extend around it, *lengthen* the ABD pad by making a wide *tape tab* at one end, with sticky sides of the tape against each other.

    4.   Tie loose ends of the Kling or Kerlix in a square knot over the restraint, and then to the bed, chair, etc., wherever needed.

Pearl (46) The Gauze Restraint

    Fold a four-by-four gauze square in half; place a cotton tie horizontally across the four-by-four, providing equal and ample length on each side to tie to the bed. Place a strip of adhesive lengthwise across the four-by-four, securing tie and allowing enough tape at each end to overlap (Figure 1-28).

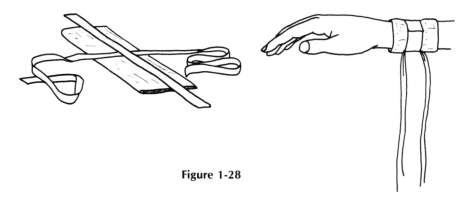

Figure 1-28

Pearl (47) Stockinette Restraints

    Stockinette can serve as light, soft restraints when needed for the toddler or infant. In addition, a safety pin can be used to secure the stockinette to the sheet for the child who is very restless (note Figure 1-29).

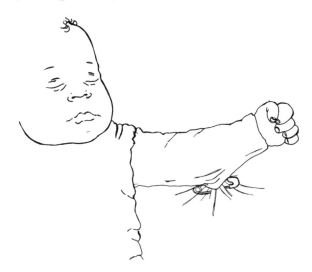

Figure 1-29

Pearl (48) Peds Diaper Restraint

To protect the infusion from accidental bumps and jars and for easy positioning of the infant, use the following restraint (see Figure 1-30). Wrap one or two diapers around the extremity which has the infusion (IV), if used in conjunction with the IV board and catheter-type needle instead of a butterfly needle. The site can be easily observed without unwrapping.
1. Diaper is folded in half or thirds.
2. Roll from ends inward.
3. Secure across the two pieces of tape.

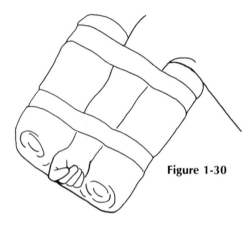

Figure 1-30

Pearl (49) An Infant Armboard and Restraint

Make an infant armboard quickly by placing two tongue depressors together (one beneath the other) and wrapping with a four-by-four gauze square. Place the infant's arm on this board (Figure 1-31, right). Restrain by placing a folded four-by-four gauze square lengthwise on the arm. Place a six-inch strip of three-inch tape (which is folded in together lengthwise) across arm and over the folded gauze square. Pin the tape edges to the bed linen (Figure 1-31, left).

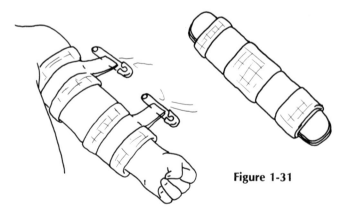

Figure 1-31

Pearl (50) Restraining the Patient on a Stretcher

When it is necessary to restrain a patient on a stretcher it is important to place the restraints across his joints (knees, elbows, etc.) rather than across soft tissue (such as his abdomen). By applying restraints across a joint, movement above and below the joint is prevented, thus preventing injury to the patient.

Another thing to remember whenever applying restraints is that the patient should be told, in advance if possible, the reason for restraints.

Pearl (51) Have a Restraint Bed Ready for Emergencies

The psychiatric unit has found it helpful to keep one bed set up at all times with leather restraints already in position. In the event that the bed is needed suddenly, wasted time and the confusion of ordering, opening, and positioning the restraints are prevented by having it ready in advance.

MINIMIZING PROBLEMS OF IMMOBILITY

In addition to encouraging mobility, the nurse has an equally important goal of *minimizing problems* associated with patients who have altered mobility for whatever reason. The following pearls will aid you in meeting this goal.

Pearl (52) Short-Tubing—Limits Mobility

Use connectors to add extra lengths of tubing. Lengthening the tubing provides for greater range of mobility (i.e., turning, repositioning, ambulating or sitting the patient up in a chair at the bedside).

Pearl (53) Wrist Strap

A strap or piece of tape can be tied about four inches below the neck of the cane or stick. Then it may be hung on the wrist when walking up stairs.

Pearl (54) The Magic of the Rubber Band

To secure drainage tubes while encouraging movement of the patient, a rubber band which overlaps the tube and is pulled through itself can be used. It is then fastened to the patient's gown or bed linens with a safety pin. The elasticity of the rubber band keeps the tube in place while providing enough flexibility for patient movement. Adhesive tape used to overlap the tube and secured with a safety pin does not allow this flexibility (Figure 1-32).

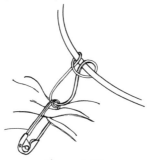

Figure 1-32

Pearl (55) The Improvised Call Light

For patients who are unable to press the call light, tape the tip of the barrel of a syringe to the call light. Any movements of the syringe barrel will depress the call button and turn on the light (Figure 1-33).

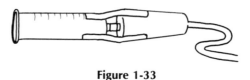

Figure 1-33

Pearl (56) Extra Water in the Tub for Buoyancy

If you fill the tub almost full of water after the patient has completed bathing, this added buoyancy makes lifting a heavy patient out of the tub easier. Protect the floor from getting wet during this maneuver.

Pearl (57) The Velcro Strip

Velcro strips can serve many useful purposes for the patient who has difficulty using his hands (e.g., they can be used in place of zippers, buttons, etc.). These can be purchased at any fabric shop.

Pearl (58) Utility Clip

In addition to serving as mop and broom holders, the household utility clip has many uses in the hospital. Three examples are the following:
1. Holding a syringe or an ampule within easy reach for the "stat" use
2. Keeping the patient's cane within reach but off the floor
3. Placing the reusable asepto syringe needed for gastric feedings

Pearl (59) A Seat in the Tub

Place a *sturdy* stool (about six to eight inches in height) to provide an elevated seat in the bathtub for patients who have trouble trying to get in and out of the tub.

Pearl (60) The Pick-up Tongs

The "helping hand" is a gadget that is like long tongs. It is used for the patient to pick up small articles from the floor without having to bend (e.g., a mother with arthritis would find it very helpful in picking up small objects off her son's bedroom floor). It can be purchased commercially.

Pearl (61) Plate Guards

Use these metal strips clipped to the edge of the plate securely. They serve to aid the patient in picking up his food, as the food can be pushed against the guard. These can be purchased commercially.

Pearl (62) The Aids for Enlarging a Key

The patient who has difficulty with fine hand movements such as are required to handle a key can 1) fit the key into a piece of cork; 2) glue it into a piece of styrofoam; or 3) wrap the head of the key securely in a piece of fabric or gauze until it is bulky and easy to manipulate.

Pearl (63) Brassieres for the Geriatric Patient

A well-supporting brassiere which hooks in the front is preferred by the elderly woman and by the woman with physical limitations in movement because it is easy to apply and remove.

Pearl (64) Rubber Band for the Lipstick

To aid the patient with limited movement of the fingers (because of arthritis, after a stroke, or any neurological disruption), twist a rubber band around the lipstick tube. This allows better grasp on the tube and makes application easier. This rubber band can also be used on combs, electric razors, etc.

Pearl (65) Push-Button Light Switches

Push-button electric power switches are easier for the person who has difficulty with prehension and weakness in the hand to control the room lighting. Place a clothes pin or a strip of heavy rubber tubing over the switch so that it will lengthen the switch for easier control.

GADGETS FOR FACILITATING MOBILITY
Pearl (66) Surgi-lift

The Surgi-lift which is shown in Figure 1-34, is used to safely transport patients from the operating room table to the postanesthesia recovery room (PARR)

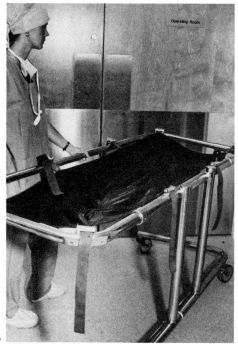

Figure 1-34

bed. It is also used in the burn unit and in transporting other patients (such as the patient with neurological dysfunction) from one bed to the other, or from a bed to a high-standing shower tub.

The major advantages of this gadget are that it 1) helps maintain physiological stability in patients who may encounter untoward alteration in vital signs from the usual transfer from bed to bed; 2) permits transportation of patient when there is limited personnel to assist with difficult transfer; and 3) is often less frightening and more comfortable to the patient.

Other helpful gadgets for patient mobility (and immobility) which we have found particularly helpful include the following:

Soft restraints, heel and elbow protectors, and numerous other helpful items by the J. T. Posey Company

Roto Rest Treatment Table (Kinetic Concepts)

Disposable bathmat

Fracture bedpan

Sleeves for armboards (Arm Hospital)

Rubber heels for walking casts (Zimmer Orthopedic)

Transport bed

Tilt-A-Bed

Span-Aide Body Positioners

Stretcher-wheelchair

Obesity bypass wheelchair

Roto-bed (Figure 1-35)

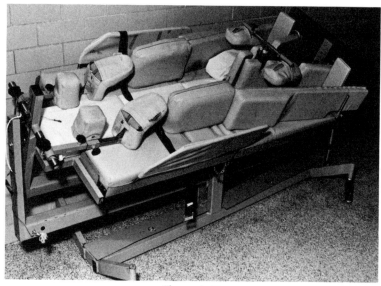

Figure 1-35

Comfort and Hygiene

Chapter two

An important part of the nursing care plan is the implementation of appropriate interventions for promoting the optimum comfort of your patient.

Appropriate nursing measures can be implemented after assessing the physical comfort needs of the patient. For instance, the nurse must consider if the patient is restless, warm and dry, in dire need of good oral hygiene, or has a disability, incision, drain, etc. that causes discomfort.

Modifications in patient care and creative improvisions which promote physical comfort of the patient are stressed in this chapter.

BATH-TIME
Pearl (1) A Genuine Bed Bath

Certainly, giving a bed bath to the patient who is unable to bathe himself takes extra time. However, this procedure, when properly planned, can be one of the most rewarding and valuable experiences for the nursing staff and the patient. What are a few of these rewards?

1. Cleanliness and decreasing potential of infection for the ill patient.
2. Soothing, relaxing comfort for the patient.
3. An opportunity for the patient to communicate and share his ideas, concerns, etc., with the staff.
4. A chance for the new patient to get better acquainted with those "strangers" who are caring for him.
5. An opportunity for the member of the nursing staff to do a thorough patient assessment, to teach the patient and to establish a better nurse-patient relationship.

So make assignments and/or organize the time allotted for bathing the patient carefully, just as you would in all aspects of patient care.

Here are a few pearls which we find make a difference between a bed bath and good bed bath.

Pearl (2) Privacy

Close the door or pull the curtains about the bed to provide privacy. Place a sign on the door or curtains that reads "Patient Bathing."

Pearl (3) Modesty

It is very important for the nursing staff to recognize that patients are truly *individuals* in their reaction to nudity, body exposure and concepts of modesty in general. Provide the very modest patient with an extra towel for covering in addition to the bath blanket to place over the breasts and/or perineum during the bath.

Pearl (4) Warmth

Prevent chilling by adjusting the thermostat, using a bath blanket, or keeping the water warm.

Pearl (5) A Good Soak

Place the patient's hands and feet in the basin when possible. This seems to make them feel more relaxed as well as provides cleanliness.

Place a towel under the basin as the extremity is being soaked. After removing the basin, the towel prevents the bed from becoming wet until the extremity is dried.

Pearl (6) Organizing

Gather at the bedside all the bath supplies, linens, pajamas, etc. needed to avoid having to leave the patient for prolonged or repeated periods of time.

Pearl (7) How to Support the Leg

Flex and support each of the patient's legs at the knee as it is soaked in the basin.

Pearl (8) Checking for Tell-tale Signs

Assess the patient for any telltale signs of skin breakdown, altered circulation, etc.

Pearl (9) Padding for the Sitz Bath

Regardless of the type of sitz bath apparatus (be it a tub, a special type of chair, etc.), it is important to adhere to certain principles. These include the promotion of comfort and exposure of the warm solution to the perineum or rectum in order for the bath to be effective. These principles are being applied when you:

1. Roll two large towels or draw sheets and place lengthwise under each thigh (see Figure 2-1).

2. Use a partially inflated rubber or plastic ring under the buttocks (Figure 2-1).

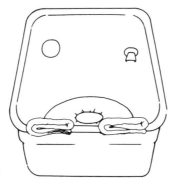

Figure 2-1

Pearl (10) A Bath Mitt Prevents Dribble

Prepare a bath mitt to eliminate dribbling and for easier management (note Figures 2-2 and 2-3). This bath mitt can be quite helpful for the patient with limited use of the fingers and paresis in the hand.

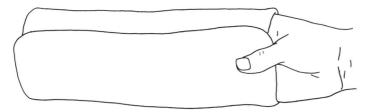

Figure 2-2

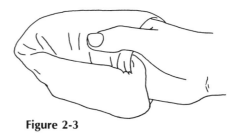

Figure 2-3

Pearl (11) Lawn Chair—A Shower Chair

The family will find it helpful to place a lawn chair in the shower for the patient who is too weak to stand to take his bath. The nurse will find that the commode chair with wheels is amenable for the same purpose, for use in the hospital.

Pearl (12) Bathing the Breasts First

Usually the nurse teaches the patient to wash her face before continuing the bath. For the lactating mother, the breasts should be bathed first. This provides more asepsis to prevent potential infection in the breasts.

Pearl (13) No Oil in the Tub

Unless the elderly person has someone to assist him in and out of the tub, oil should not be placed in the bath water. It creates a *very slippery* tub in which the patient can easily fall.

Pearl (14) Bathe as Necessary

Bathing the elderly patient daily is not always necessary. In fact it can produce dry skin since the sebaceous glands slow down as the person grows older.

However, while this is sound practice for the well elderly person, the nurse must use discretion in evaluating the need for each individual elderly patient to be bathed on a daily basis. (For instance, if he has problems such as incontinence, febrile episodes, or "night sweats," then a daily bath is important.) Also, recall that while a daily bath is prevalent among middle-class Americans, this is not always the custom in other cultures or countries. Therefore, this custom must be assessed as well.

Pearl (15) Shaving Made Easier

Apply these helpful tips to prevent nicks and cuts and for faster, easier shaving of the patient.
1. Apply a creamy lotion generously and shave.
2. Use back and forth movements with the razor but do not *lift* the razor until ready to rinse each time.
3. Keep skin pulled tautly as you shave the patient.
4. Provide a mirror if you are shaving a man's beard so that he may feel more relaxed as he observes.

Pearl (16) Kelly Pad for Shampooing

When you have a patient on bedrest who needs a shampoo, simply place a Kelly pad under the patient's head and neck. Tuck the ends of the pad into a large bath basin which is placed on a chair or in a "kick pail," with casters on the floor.

Other similar methods can be improvised if a Kelly pad is not accessible to you. (For example, use a large sheet of plastic such as a large trash bag which has been cut and opened out completely.) Roll the plastic bag with a towel or newspaper inside the folds to simulate a Kelly pad.

Pearl (17) Bathing Agents for the Elderly

Use Castile liquid soap, oil (e.g., Keri oil) or baby oil in the bath water to help prevent dry skin in the elderly patient.

MAINTAINING SKIN INTEGRITY
Pearl (18) The Good Old-Fashioned Backrub

As a finishing touch to the bed bath, to promote relaxation in an anxious patient who cannot sleep, and for many other reasons, the backrub is hard to beat.

The backrub is as beneficial today as it was in the past. A backrub which is properly administered promotes comfort, relaxation and a sense of well-being and of receiving personalized individual care from the staff and stimulates circulation to the skin.

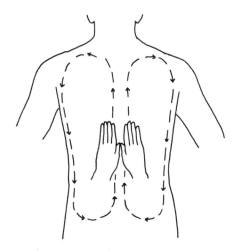

Figure 2-4

It can foster better communication. For example, the preop patient who is anxious and restless on the last evening before surgery will often share his concern with the nursing staff member during this time, as the backrub is being given.

However, while it is a simple procedure, we find the following illustrated method effective and safe. Give the backrub without rushing. You and your patient must be in comfortable positions.

1. Adjust the bed to the correct height for you. Have the patient turn on his side so that his back is toward you. (When possible avoid *alcohol*, as it causes drying of the skin; and avoid talc—this powder collects as tiny lumps on skin wet with perspiration and can lead to skin breakdown.)

2. Apply a generous amount of lanolin lotion to your hands. (Avoid squirting this cold lotion directly onto the patient's back.) Rub hands slightly to warm the lotion, or place lotion bottle in the warm bath water.

3. Begin (as illustrated in Figure 2-4), with palms flat and hands side by side at the lower back, and rub on the lotion in an upward-outward motion returning to the lower back.

4. Use good body mechanics and a "rocking to and fro" movement as you rub the patient's back.

Should there be excess lotion, *pat* skin dry.

Pearl (19) Cornstarch for the Bedpan

Dust the bedpan with cornstarch for easier placement under the patient's buttocks. This prevents the bedpan from sticking to the skin, thus eliminating skin breakdown and patient discomfort.

Pearl (20) Chux to Pad Casts

Use Chux to pad dry casts (for the thigh, pelvis, or body casts) to prevent fecal and urinary drainage from soiling the cast.

Pearl (21) Hair Dryer Used on Cool Setting

1. A hair dryer dries skin fully and quickly around stomas while changing the pouch. Dry skin increases adherence of the pouch.
2. For diaphoretic patients prone to decubiti, heat rash, etc., put the hair dryer near the bed and let it blow continuously on the patient.
3. For incontinent patients let the hair dryer blow on buttocks between cleaning. This helps prevent maceration of skin.

Pearl (22) Protective Covering for Heat/Cold Apparatus

Regardless of the type of heat or cold device (be it a hypothermal blanket, a heating pad, an ice collar) a protective cloth covering (pillowcase, towel, bath blanket) should be placed between the pad and the skin of the patient. This prevents irritation and excoriation of the skin, as well as being more comfortable.

Pearl (23) Plastic Briefs and Chux

Two devices which are helpful in the care of the female patient who has the problem of urinary incontinence are:

1. *Commercially available plastic briefs* which holds sanitary (super absorbent) napkins, and;
2. *Improvised briefs from Chux* (note Figure 2-5).

Step 1.   Fold a Chux (incontinent pad) into a triangle, securing the folded edge of one corner with nonallergic tape.

Step 2.   Fold a second Chux in the same manner, and tape.

Step 3.   Overlap one taped end of the Chux inside the other for extra thickness and better fit in the crotch.

Step 4.   Apply two strips of nonallergic tape, which are backtaped inside the Chux, at the anterior and posterior portions of the perineal area. These strips of tape will serve to secure the sanitary napkin in place. (Be sure to leave enough tape that is nonbacked at the end of each strip so that it will adhere as it overlaps to the exterior side of the Chux.)

Step 5.   The triangular-shaped Chux are pinned at the waist and at the crotch.

These improvised briefs can be adjusted to fit the individual's pelvic contour. In addition, the patient or nurse can change the peri-pads (sanitary napkins) as necessary by simply unpinning the Chux that overlaps at the perineum.

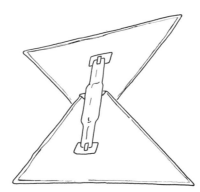

Figure 2-5

ORAL HYGIENE
Pearl (24) Mineral Oil to Lips

For the mouth-breather or for most patients with dry lips, apply a thin coating of mineral oil to the lips.

Pearl (25) No Moistened Sponge for Dry Mouth

Never use small sponges or the like when moistening the dry mouth and lips of the patients (note Figure 2-6). This is particularly crucial for the nurse in caring for patients who are not fully alert or who are uncooperative (e.g., the patient who is still drowsy from analgesics or anesthetics or who is confused). Use a *towel* in which one end is slightly damp (note Figure 2-7). This way you can keep a safe grasp on the towel, thus preventing any inadvertent airway obstruction caused by the failure to retrieve a small sponge.

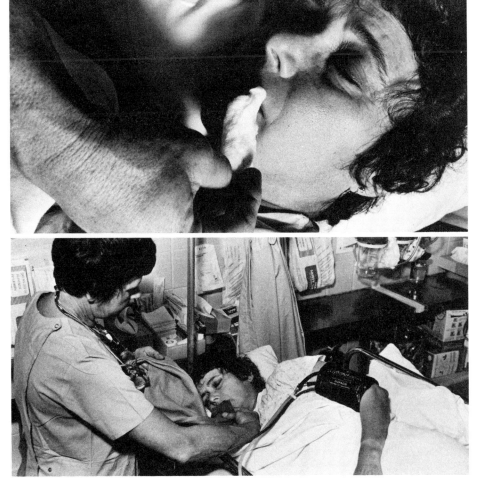

Figure 2-6 (top), **Figure 2-7** (bottom)

Pearl (26) Safe Mouth Care

To give thorough mouth care to intubated or confused patients, or to a patient with a poor cough reflex, use a suction catheter or oral suction.

Place the suction in the mouth toward the back of the throat, suction out secretions, and then *with the catheter still in place,* squirt mouthwash into the mouth, irrigating well, while applying suction. This prevents the patient from swallowing or aspirating the mouthwash.

Pearl (27) Dentures—Care and Cleaning

Dentures can be cleaned with commercial products prepared for that purpose or by placing in a cup of water with approximately 1 ml of bleach added. "Dakins," a bleach-type solution, is often supplied by pharmacies. Household baking soda can also be used as a dentifrice.

Prevent accidentally dropping and breaking dentures. When rinsing dentures do not hold under the faucet with rapid flowing water, unless they are held close to a basin which is placed below the faucet in the lavatory.

Provide a denture cup which is properly labeled with the correct identification.

Pearl (28) This Butterdish Holds No Butter

Used plastic butterdishes containing a little water are excellent for storage of the patient's denture; they will not break and the lid helps prevent spills and is easy to apply and remove. These dishes can be washed with soap and water and dried daily or discarded for another.

Other aspects of personal hygiene, changing the gown and "making the bed" are *important* comfort measures which are, in nursing, too often called simply "routine daily care."

SKIN SAVERS IN DRESSING CHANGES

Pearls of nursing care are needed to promote comfort while ministering therapeutic procedures.

Pearl (29) Folding Tape Edges

When applying tape, fold the ends slightly (Figure 2-8). This will aid in the removal of the tape and avoid potential trauma from scratching or pinching of the skin when the edges of the tape are not easily grasped.

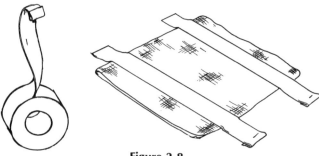

Figure 2-8

Pearl (30) Use of Dressenet

This is a new fabric resembling a slightly elasticized fishnet which comes in various sizes. It is tubular in shape and can slip over torso or extremities to keep dressings intact without using tape.

Pearl (31) Paper Tape—A Skin Saver

When tape is needed to secure a dressing, paper tape is less irritating than adhesive tape.

Pearl (32) Protecting the Skin Around the Trach Site

Two common methods which can be safely applied to prevent irritation of the skin and aid in preventing infection from stagnant accumulated mucous on the skin about the trach are shown in the following illustrations (Figures 2-9 and 2-10).

1. A four-by-four gauze sponge is cut to center of sponge. Then each side of cut stitched securely to prevent loose frayed edges which could be aspirated. Our CSR supplies these in the trach-care kits.

2. An alternate method is to take a four-by-four gauze sponge, open it to a four-by-eight size, and fold it lengthwise. Grasp one corner on the fold-side and invert at center. Then do the same with the opposite corner on the fold. This will provide a protective dressing that is also safe from ragged edges at the trach site.

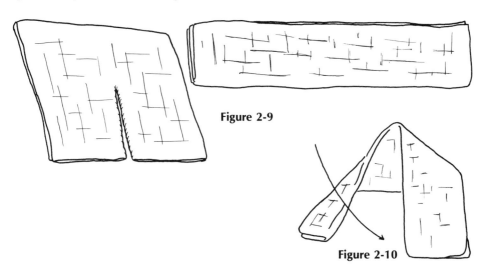

Figure 2-9

Figure 2-10

PERSONAL ITEMS AND CLOTHING
Pearl (33) Shopping at the Bedside

Small personal items such as lipstick, toothpaste, stationery, and combs can be purchased by the patient at the bedside if a small cart is organized with such items and brought around to the rooms.

The volunteers should always report in at the nurse's station before pushing the cart to the various rooms. The nurse or unit secretary can advise them on which rooms should be included on the shopping cart rounds that day.

Pearl (34) Bib for the Patient

Your patient who has difficulty feeding himself, due to paresis, weakness, muscular tremors, etc., needs to have his gown or clothes protected with a bib. These can be improvised from a hand towel, Chux or drawsheet. It is most disconcerting to the patient and his family to find that he has soiled himself from spilling food because he failed to use such a simple object as the bib.

Pearl (35) The Easy Open Sleeve

Removing the hospital gown from a patient with an infusion or cast can be a time-consuming and tedious process, not to mention a discomfort to the patient and a possible disruption of the infusion.

The following are two suggestions to help in removing the gown safely and easily:

1. Place gowns on the patients which have ties, "snaps," velcro strips, etc. as sleeve closures rather than the conventional seam.
2. When the usual hospital gowns with seams in the sleeves are used, apply the following procedure for *easier removal of the gown:*
   a. Untie the gown at the neckline.
   b. Remove the gown from the extremity which is free of the infusion, dressing or cast.
   c. Pull the gown gently off the extremity which has the infusion or cast, etc.
   d. If it is an infusion in the arm, then pass the infusion bag up through the sleeve from the distal end of the sleeve, removing it from the proximal portion (shoulder opening) of the sleeve.
   e. Reverse the process when applying a gown. Some staff members find this procedure easier to do by thinking of the IV as an extension of the patient's arm.

Pearl (36) Removing Clothes from a Patient in the ER

Effective treatment of a patient in the emergency room often demands that clothing be removed. To easily remove clothes from a patient who is lying flat and unable to help himself, stand behind the head of the patient and raise his arms all the way above his head.

Then pull the shirt or dress and any underclothes off with one motion. Of course this is after loosening any buttons or fasteners.

Pearl (37) PJ's and the Modest Patient

For your patient who cannot stand up to put on his pajamas, but needs assistance, use this simple approach:

1. Loosen the top sheet at the foot of the bed.
2. Reach under the topsheet and slip each pajama leg (which is gathered in your hand) over each foot.
3. Slide the pajamas upward to the knees.

4. The pj's should be within easy reach for the patient to complete dressing.

Soiled pj's can be removed by reversing the process—beginning with the patient reaching under the sheet and pushing them to his knees, etc.

Pearl (38) Removing That *Tight* Ring

A ring that has been worn for quite some time, or a ring on an edematous extremity can become tight enough to be difficult to remove. Here is a really intriguing little tip (Figure 2-11).

1. Wrap a piece of string tightly around the finger immediately distal to the ring.
2. Pull the ring forward until it meets the string.
3. Wrap the string again, moving it again distal from the ring but still very close to the ring.
4. Proceed in this fashion until the ring is removed.

(Here's how it works: the string pushes down the skin in front of the ring allowing it to move forward. By advancing the string you can pull the ring off a little at a time.)

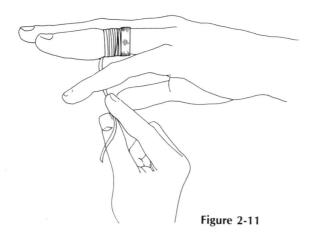

Figure 2-11

Pearl (39) Temporary Scuffs

Save the large heavy duty wrapping from sterile packages, which are processed in sterile processing. These can be used to make temporary slippers or scuffs. These are much better than the old newspaper slipper, as these wrappings are readily available and there is no newsprint to rub off as it comes in contact with the moisture and body heat of the feet. Make these paper scuffs the same way you have probably observed children doing so for fun (note Figures 2-12, 2-13, 2-14, and 2-15).

The steps involved are to:

1. Fold the wrapping in half lengthwise.
2. Fold the lower end toward the upper end of the wrapping, making a center fold.

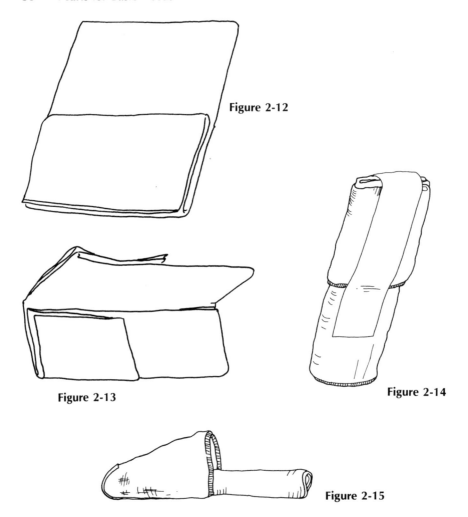

Figure 2-12

Figure 2-13

Figure 2-14

Figure 2-15

3. Turn the edge of the topsheet down to the center fold (Figure 2-12). Turn the wrapping over.
4. Now fold from side to side in thirds, creasing the folds (Figure 2-13).
5. Tuck the entire left side into the right cuff.
6. Fold the free end of the cuff inward. Reinforce the edges and sole of the scuff with tape (Figure 2-14).
7. After turning the scuff over, slip your hand into the cuff and gently raise the toe of the scuff (Figure 2-15).
    Keep a supply of these scuffs on hand in small, medium and large sizes.

Pearl (40) Lighted Magnifying Glass

Adequate lighting as well as corrective lenses helps the older person with failing eyesight. There is a small size hand magnifying glass which has a light. This is helpful in reading small print such as advertisements and the telephone directory. These are sold over the counter in local drug stores.

Pearl (41) Rubber Band for Spectacles

Use a large thick rubber band to attach to glasses that do not fit snugly enough (note Figure 2-16). The rubber band connects one side of the frames to the other as it crosses behind the neck. Similar commercial devices which clip on can be purchased.

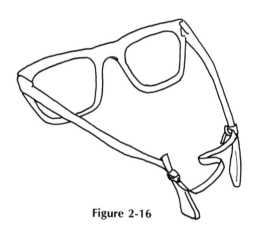

Figure 2-16

MAKING THE BED
Pearl (42) Admire and Tug

Teach your staff to give a tug to those clean top linens as they pause to admire that "perfect" bed which they have just completed making.

Where and how to tug? Grasp the center of the top linens at the foot of the bed and tug gently to loosen these linens without untucking them.

Why tug? This provides more space for movement of the patient's feet and legs. This simple maneuver is particularly important for the bedridden patient in helping to prevent footdrop.

Pearl (43) How to Put on a Pillowcase

Here is the quickest and easiest way to put a pillowcase on a pillow. (Note: this also promotes infection control since the pillow is not held against the nurse's uniform.)

1. With one hand grasp the short seam of the pillow case.
2. With the other hand hold the pillow.
3. While continuing to hold the pillowcase, also grasp the pillow with the same hand.
4. Smooth down the pillowcase (see Figures 2-17 and 2-18).

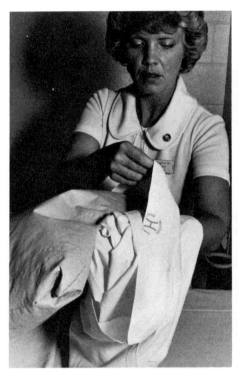 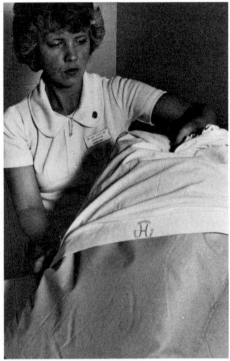

Figure 2-17   Figure 2-18

Pearl (44) Fitting the Flat Sheet

Thin mattresses with nonabsorbent covers may be the way the world is going, but they certainly do not make it any easier to make a tight bed, particularly with flat sheets. A restless patient can ruin his freshly made bed in no time. Tying the sheet at the foot and head of the bed solves this problem nicely.

Pearl (45) Make the Traction Bed from *Top to Bottom*

The patient who is in traction can assist with his bed-making and thereby feel more comfortable by using his overhead trapeze while the nurse makes his bed from top to bottom. The procedure is as follows and may involve one to three nurses, depending upon the strength of the patient (and the skill of the nurses). (Note Figures 2-19 and 2-20.)

1. Center the sheet at the top of the bed.
2. Tuck the top of the sheet under the mattress.
3. Fan-fold the sheet so that it is all at the top of the bed.
4. Lift the patient's shoulders (or have him lift with his trapeze), and pull the sheet down as far as it will go.
5. Lift the patient's hips (or have him lift them) and pull the sheet over the mattress.
6. Tuck and/or tie the sheet under the mattress.
7. Have the patient lift his hips again to apply a drawsheet or sheepskin to the bed.
8. Now that the bed is made, make the patient comfortable.

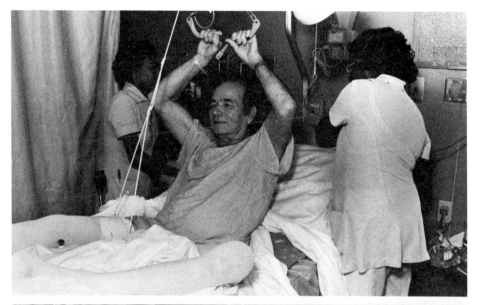

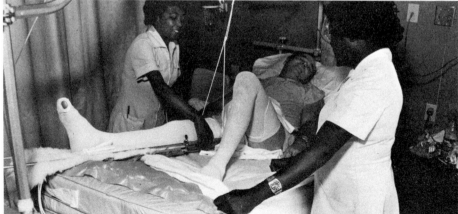

Figure 2-19 (top), **Figure 2-20** (bottom)

COMFORT MEASURES FOR THE PATIENT WITH THE NASOGASTRIC TUBE

Important aspects of nursing care of the patient with a nasogastric (NG) tube include the following pearls.

Pearl (46) Oral Hygiene

Provide good oral hygiene. Lemon drops, Gatorgum, peppermint, etc., are refreshing and help relieve thirst in these patients who cannot have oral fluids.

Pearl (47) Clean Nares

Clean the nostrils, particularly where the tube is located, daily and prn.

1. An applicator, moistened with diluted hydrogen peroxide removes mucous crusts and other dried secretions including dried blood.

2. After cleaning around the tube in the nares, apply a water-soluble lubricant or a small amount of bacteriostatic ointment with an applicator.

Pearl (48) Rotate Tube

Rotate the tube gently at intervals to prevent excoriation and discomfort from pressure of the tube in one location. Be careful to avoid pulling or pushing on the tube, as this could cause displacement. (Occasionally, the patient will also complain of severe tenderness in his throat near the eustacian tube. Rotating the tube often relieves this tenderness and discomfort.)

Pearl (49) Displacement of the Tape

Should the tape which secures the placement of the tube become soiled or begin to loosen, remove the tape, clean the skin on the nose and reapply with new tape.

DECREASING DISCOMFORT

Pearl (50) Prop the Foot—On What?

The patient has to have his foot elevated? You are out of foot stools? A chair is too high? Time to improvise! Put a pillow on a small trash basket and you have made a nice, soft stool that is just the right height.

Pearl (51) Gas Pains

A common complaint of patients as the intestines resume functioning following abdominal surgery is the discomfort of gas pains.

Measures which aid in the relief of this problem include: a) ambulating the patient; b) changing the positions of the patient in bed; c) loosening constricting clothing; d) providing privacy, particularly when the patient is on the bedpan or the commode (This is very important since the patient will often endure the discomfort of gas pains rather than be embarrassed by trying to expel the flatus when others are present.); and e) inserting a rectal tube. It is also helpful to use the following additional measures when a rectal tube is inserted.

1. Place a Chux under the patient to prevent any soiling of the bed linens. Be sure to tell the patient the Chux is in place, to eliminate his worry over possibly soiling the linens. It also aids in his ability to relax and try to expel the flatus.

2. Help eliminate unpleasant odor in the room by placing the external end of the rectal tube into a small plastic bag through a slit made in the top of a stool specimen container.

3. Keep deodorizer available in the room.

Pearl (52) The Bellevue Bridge

A scrotal support can be made from two pieces of three-inch wide tape. Place a shorter piece of the tape (adhesive side to adhesive side) across the patient's thighs. Place a small folded cloth on the tape, elevating the scrotum. (The Bellevue Bridge can only be used for patients on bedrest and who are not restless.) A piece of steri-drape can be substituted for the adhesive.

CARING FOR THE OBESE PATIENT

Hetercene Turner Dee, R.T.N. III (Head Nurse of the third floor ambulant wing, Shands Teaching Hospital) has developed several practical items which are particularly helpful in the care of obesity by-pass patients. Note Figure 2-21 for an example of a few of such gadgets. Their descriptions follow.

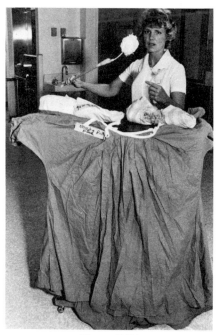

Figure 2-21

Pearl (53) Obesity By-pass Arm Extender

This mop is improvised from a basic glass and dish mop manufactured by Empire, Inc., Port Chester, N.Y. Similar basic glass and dish mops can be purchased locally.

The obesity by-pass patient has problems reaching to clean the anal, vaginal and groin area. The arm is not long enough to reach, especially postoperatively.

A nursing staff member was called often to clean the patients (as many as 15 times per day) according to severity of the diarrhea. The patients were mortified with embarrassment and frequently "dissolved in tears." The nursing staff when very busy was impatient.

Solution to problems: Three and a half years ago this nurse made the arm extender from mops. Patients and nursing staff were delighted. Patients could use the same type of mop for reaching back areas during showers or baths.

The arm extender is introduced to all preop obesity by-pass patients almost immediately after admission and during preop teaching.

Hospital stores now supply the mops and other needed materials especially for the obese patient.

Pearl (54) Obesity By-pass Gowns and Robes

Because of the size of these patients, no usual hospital gowns or robes would fit. Three and a half years ago, the R.T.N. III on our ambulant unit at Shands Teaching Hospital asked linen service to make special gowns and robes. The unit had no budget money available for this, so old pastel sheets were used.

Later when more gowns and robes were needed, they used old drape material for robes and unbleached muslin for the gowns. These are soft and very durable. The need was to have a style big enough to accommodate a 200 to 650 pound person. The nurse designed a style that was attractive and practical and would look good on a male or female patient.

Pearl (55) Description of the Style of Robe

Style of robe: pleats, unstitched, to open out for any size patient. The front completely overlaps to give a double front if needed or close to a smaller size. Ties are used for closing. There is an opening in the back for accessibility for examinations, procedures, x-rays, etc.

IV Therapy, Nutrition and Hydration

Chapter three

Adequate nutrition and hydration are essential needs that must be met to achieve or maintain homeostasis in the patient. Malnutrition, obesity, dehydration and over-hydration are common problems which the nurse encounters as she cares for the patient. The nurse has a major role in collaborating and working with the nutritionist, physician and other members of the health team in combating and preventing these problems.

The nurse must consider those factors which alter the fluid and nutritional needs of the patient. Some of these factors are body size, activity level, age, sex, illness, and environment.

For instance, it is obvious that the lactating mother, the feeble infant, the patient on isolation or bedrest, the patient with a gastrostomy tube, etc., all require modifications for adequate nutrition and hydration.

In this chapter you will find pearls that suggest alternative interventions in meeting the nutritional and fluid needs of the patient. Pearls are cited for such specific considerations as:
1. Accurate fluid intake
2. Alternate routes of feeding and fluid intake
3. Enticing the patient to eat
4. Intravenous therapy

PEARLS FOR STARTING THE INFUSION
Pearl (1) Use Nondominant Extremity

Ascertain if the patient is right-handed or left-handed. You can provide greater range of mobility by using the nondominant extremity for the infusion site.

Pearl (2) The Right Location

Although veins often appear easier to enter at such locations as the joints (e.g., brachial fossa), this limits the mobility of the extremity, which is more prone to injury unless securely immobilized.

Pearl (3) The Tourniquet Can Wait

Place the extremity in a dependent position as you assess for the appropriate site. This should be done prior to applying a tourniquet. (Prolonged use of the tourniquet should always be avoided.) Instructing the patient to open and close his hand (pumping of the hand) while the extremity is dependent also facilitates venous distention.

Pearl (4) No Slapping

The practice of slapping the extremity serves no real purpose but frightens the patient unnecessarily and should be discouraged.

Pearl (5) Bevel Up versus Bevel Down

The advantage of having the bevel of the needle up when inserting into the vein is that it allows earlier detection of infiltration than with the bevel-down approach. This is the usual approach preferred when inserting the needle into a vein that is much larger than the diameter of the needle (Figure 3-1).

When inserting the needle into a vein that is approximately the same size as the diameter of the needle, it is best to insert with the bevel down. The advantages are that it prevents collapse of the vein wall over the needle lumen and prevents possible perforation of the posterior walls of the vessel (Figure 3-2).

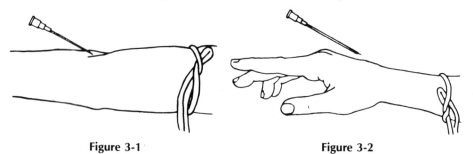

Figure 3-1   Figure 3-2

Pearl (6) Shaving the Site

Too often the most painful part of the infusion procedure is removing tape from a hairy extremity. So shave the area prior to starting the infusion.

Pearl (7) Begin Distally

Since the first attempt to start the infusion is not always successful, it may become necessary to make another insertion. First select a distal site, in order to have access to a more proximal site on the same vein, should a second attempt be needed. (Remember venous blood flows *toward* the heart, and after an earlier proximal site is attempted, the distal site will not be useful because of disruption of the venous route on that vessel.)

Pearl (8) One Stick—Two Steps

While there is *only one actual insertion site*, two steps should be considered when inserting the needle: step 1 involves puncturing the skin and step 2 involves threading the needle into the vein. To avoid passing through the vein as you puncture the skin, which is tougher tissue than the vein, do not start the insertion over the vein. Instead, begin skin puncture slightly adjacent to and about one-quarter inch away, while holding the needle at a 30° to 45° angle (Figure 3-3). Then, once through the skin, lower the needle parallel to the skin and aligned with the vein and thread the needle into the vein (Figure 3-4).

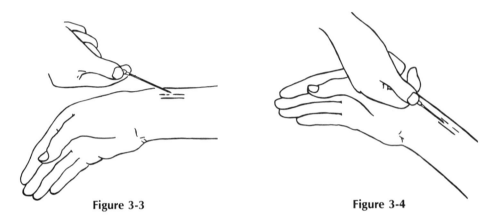

Figure 3-3   Figure 3-4

Pearl (9) Reaching the Flow-Rate Adaptor

Have all the equipment in readiness for the infusion at the bedside. Clear the tubing of air. Move the flow-rate adjustor near the distal end of the tubing and make certain it is completely turned off. This eliminates infiltration of the tissue with fluid as you insert the needle. It also prevents unnecessary movement and delay in having to reach and search for the adaptor when it is time to start the fluid flow.

Once the solution has started infusing, keep the needle or catheter in the vein. To do so involves using ingenuity in improvising measures that will stabilize the needle or catheter at the infusion site without injury. Also, provide as much mobility as possible for that particular patient's situation.

The following pearls should be considered:

Pearl (10) Stabilize Promptly

Immediately following insertion into the vein, keep one hand stabilizing the needle or catheter at all times to prevent displacement until it is secured by other means (i.e., tape, etc.).

Pearl (11) Securing the Hub

Using a strip of one-inch tape (three inches in length), place the tape (adhesive side up) under the hub. Take each end of the tape and cross over the hub, securing it to the skin (note Figure 3-5). A cotton ball or alcohol wipe should be placed under the hub to prevent irritation of the skin.

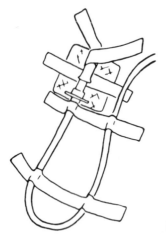

Figure 3-5

When placing a dressing or tape over the infusion site, leave the junction where the tubing connects with the hub uncovered so that it can be disconnected without difficulty to change the tubing when necessary.

Pearl (12) Loop the Tubing

Make a loop in the tubing (without occluding the flow) as illustrated in Figure 3-5, to prevent tension on and inadvertent displacement of the needle.

When stabilizing and securing the IV (infusion), provide for as much visualization of the tubing and extremity as possible in order to observe for any problems at the insertion site or in the tubing (e.g., backflow, air, etc.), as well as the condition of the patient's extremity. This *can be done without the use of an overabundance of tape.* Velcro strips, gauze restraints, armboards, and backtaping can be used in a variety of ways to meet these requirements.

Pearl (13) Gauze Restraints

Gauze restraints (see chapter on mobility) certainly save wear and tear of the patient's skin when properly applied. These can be altered to fit over any extremity or armboard.

Pearl (14) Backtaping

When attaching a patient's arm to an IV board, why not back the tape? Tear two pieces of adhesive tape, one several inches shorter than the other. Center the shorter piece on the longer one with their adhesive sides together. You now have a piece of tape which is adhesive on the ends, where you need it to be, but not in the middle, where you don't. Using tape in this fashion to fix an extremity to an IV armboard avoids unnecessary trauma to the skin and makes removal of the armboard when the IV is discontinued much easier and less painful.

Pearl (15) Tape—A Restraint or Tourniquet?

When applying tape around an extremity avoid overlapping the ends of the tape (particularly adhesive tape). Always leave a small margin of skin free from tape.

Why? Should swelling occur as a result of position change or from infiltration of the infusion solution, the tape ends which are overlapped can constrict the blood flow like a tourniquet, causing trauma, ischemia and pain. Unlike the skin, tape provides no elasticity.

Pearl (16) Use of the Armboard

When applying armboards, provide for extension of the board above and below the joint to be stabilized.

For instance at the elbow, when the basilic or cephalic veins are used, place the armboard from approximately two inches above the elbow, extended to the fingers. Or, for instance, when the infusion site is more distal in the extremity, it may be only necessary to use a short board which extends from two inches above the insertion site to the fingers (note Figures 3-6 and 3-7).

When possible, provide for extension and flexion of the fingers. Place restraints as needed across the hand, leaving the thumb free and the fingers movable. Place a rolled washcloth under the fingers to aid in normal positioning of the hand.

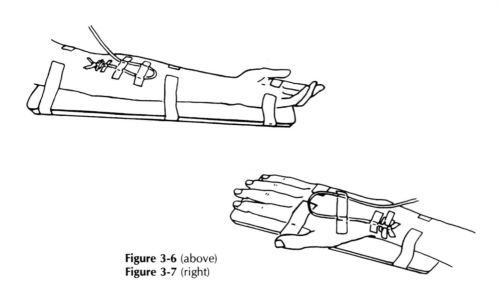

Figure 3-6 (above)
Figure 3-7 (right)

Pearl (17) Inserting the Intravenous Catheter

After inserting the needle of an intravenous catheter into the vein, as soon as a flashback of blood is obtained, start passing the catheter. If resistance is met, stop passing the catheter and turn the IV fluid on at a very rapid rate. Usually the force of the fluid gently eases the catheter into the patient's vein.

This method may save the patient from multiple insertions for IV sites. Sometimes too hasty entry into the vein results in infiltration.

TOURNIQUETS—APPLICATION AND IMPROVISIONS
Pearl (18) Applying the Tourniquet

Place the center of the tourniquet under the extremity (note Figure 3-8). Grasp each end with one hand, pulling tautly. Stretching the tourniquet, fold the looped end of the tourniquet under the other end. A tourniquet applied in such a manner can be loosened with one hand by the nurse. This is particularly useful when trying to keep the infusion needle in the vein while needing to release the tourniquet prior to opening the flow-adaptor gauge.

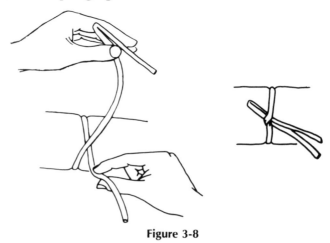

Figure 3-8

Pearl (19) Improvised Tourniquet

Strips of Penrose drain make excellent soft, pliable tourniquets. Blood pressure cuffs can be inflated and used as tourniquets also. When using blood pressure cuffs as tourniquets, place the cuff three to four inches above the intended insertion site. Inflate the cuff until the pulse, which is immediately distal to the cuff disappears. Then release the cuff pressure slowly until the pulse is barely perceptible. This slows venous return increasing local venous distention without obliterating local arterial circulation.

Of course tourniquets can be fashioned from many other materials, including strips of torn clothing, gauze strips, handkerchieves, etc., when needed.

PEARLS FOR REGULATING THE INFUSION

The rate of flow will vary depending on the fluid needs of the patient, the height of the solution bag or bottle, amount of fluid in the container, gauge needle, viscosity of the solution, position of the patient, and the adjustment of the flow-rate clamp. While the rate is usually ordered by the physician in terms of desired amount per hour, it is important that the nurse regulate the flow to achieve the rate as precisely as possible. Adjusting the flow rate based on a mere glance or observation relying on the illogical assumption that with "experience" one no longer needs to compute the flow rate mathematically is a haphazard approach. Determining the number of drops per minute will achieve a more accurate flow rate and thereby better meet the fluid needs of the patient.

Pearl (20) How to Compute Drops Per Minute

Each company (e.g., Abbott, Travenol, etc.) lists the number of drops (gtts) per milliliter (ml) with the accompanying infusion fluid administration set.

Generally the nurse will encounter one of three flow rates per drip chamber:
1. The drip chamber that infuses 10 gtts (drops)/ml.
2. The drip chamber that infuses 15 gtts (drops)/ml.
3. The drip chamber that infuses 60 gtts (drops)/ml.

Rule #1 Computing Drops–Simplified Method

Table 3-1A. When dealing with a drip chamber that infuses 10 gtts per ml, simply divide the number of ml ordered per hour by 6 (i.e., rate ordered: infuse 120 ml/hr; 120 divided by 6 = 20 gtts per minute or 5 gtts every 15 seconds).

The rationale for the computations and simplified method using Rule #1 cited in Table 3-1A is the following: There are 120 ml to be infused every hour. By multiplying this number (120) by 10 (the number of drops determined by the particular type of infusion set), you will find 1200 gtts are to be infused in one hour or 60 minutes; 1200 gtts is divided by 60 minutes, or 120 gtts divided by 6 minutes, which gives 20 gtts per minute.

Table 3-1B. Computing Drops—Lengthy Method

120 x 10=1200 gtts/ml
1200 gtts divided by 60 minutes =
120 gtts divided by 6 = 20 gtts/min

Rule #2 Computing Drops—Simplified Method

Table 3-2A. When using a drip chamber which infuses 15 gtts per ml simply divide the number of ml ordered per hour by 4 (i.e., rate ordered: infuse 120 ml per hour; 120 divided by 4 = 30 gtts per minute or 12 to 13 gtts every 15 seconds).

The rationale for the computations cited in Table 3-2A is the following: There are 120 ml to be infused every hour. By multiplying this number (120) by 15 (the number of drops determined by the particular type of infusion set) you will find 1800 gtts are to be infused in one hour (or 60 minutes), 1800 gtts divided by 60 = 180 divided by 6, or 30 gtts every minute.

Table 3-2B. Computing Drops—Lengthy Method

120 x 15 = 1800 gtts/hr
1800 divided by 60 minutes = 30 gtts per minute

Rule #3. Computing Drops—Lengthy Method

Table 3-3. When using a drop chamber (such as the mini or micro drip) while infusing 60 "mini" gtts per minute. Ordered rate: infuse fluid at 120 ml per hr; 120 ml times 60 (number of mini drops = 7200) mini gtts per hour or 120 mini gtts per minute or 30 mini gtts every 15 seconds.

Consequently as you will note from the computations cited in Table 3-3, if the drip chamber has a mini (micro) dropper flow at the rate of infusion, you simply infuse the mini drops per minute at the same numeral of fluid cited in the order. In other words, no computation is necessary.

Whenever in doubt of regulating fluids, have someone check your computations and assist in adjusting the actual flow rate.

Pearl (21) Timing the Drops

When regulating the infusion rate, *place your watch at eye level* behind the drip chamber. This facilitates counting the drops more accurately by eliminating the need to look away or down at your watch (note Figure 3-9).

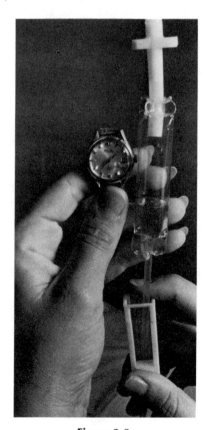

Figure 3-9

Pearl (22) Regulating Two Infusions into the Same Infusion Site

There is an increase in the administering of medications (such as antibiotics) intravenously over a short time period (usually 30 minutes to one hour). Often the patient has a heparin lock or a maintenance IV solution infusing. The short-term infusion (such as medication) can be infused into the same insertion site by use of a three-way stopcock, a "Y" connector or "piggy-back" (Figures 3-10, 3-11, and 3-12). Lower the maintenance infusion bag below the level of the short-term infusion solution bag (see Figure 3-13). This can be attained by using a Kerlix (gauze strip) or a metal hanger adapter provided by companies specifically for this purpose. This height alteration provides for more accurate infusion of the short-term solution while keeping the maintenance fluid also infusing. Whenever in doubt of potential over-hydration by such a set-up, collaborate with the physician prior to its use.

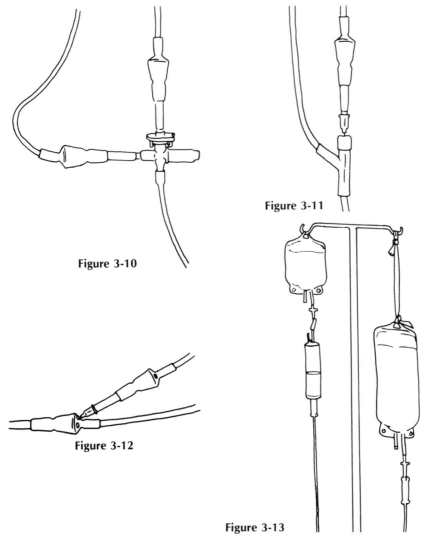

Figure 3-11

Figure 3-10

Figure 3-12

Figure 3-13

Pearl (23) Use of Extra Length of IV Tubing

Extra length of IV tubing provides extra range of mobility for the patient and also serves as a safety measure in preventing an air embolus—particularly when several solutions are infusing simultaneously and in the event that the patient elevates the extremity above the level of the right atrium.

Pearl (24) Handy Checklist—Infusion Is
Or Is Not Flowing Adequately

1. Is it due to a patient position problem (i.e., patient lying on the tubing, patient's arm flexed)?
2. Is the tubing connected at the hub? (Movement of a restless patient can pull the tubing apart.)
3. Is the tape or restraint too tight? Is there swelling?
4. Is the solution container empty? (Has it "run dry"?)
5. Does the infusion pole need to be raised to a higher level? (This is often the case as the amount of fluid decreases in the container.)
6. Is the clamp (flow-rate adaptor) open enough or is it "shut-off"? (This is one you should especially note when the patient has been transferred from one area to another.)
7. Is the needle or catheter still in the vein? Check by lowering the fluid container below the level of the patient's bed and squeezing once on the rubber bulb. If

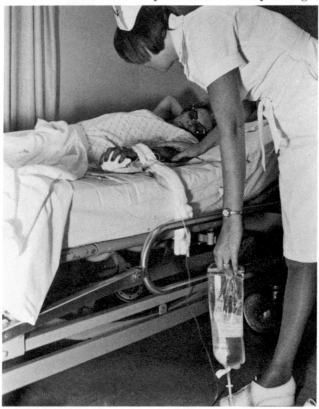

Figure 3-14

blood returns, it is in the vein. Quickly return the container to the IV pole (at a level above the needle site), to prevent clotting in the tubing (Figure 3-14).

8. Is the air filter plugged?

9. Will the IV flow if the hub is slightly elevated? If so, place a cotton ball under the hub. This maneuver is helpful when the anterior wall of the vessel has collapsed against the bevel.

10. Will the IV flow if you squeeze the rubber bulb? Occasionally a tiny clot has formed over the bevel or the anterior vessel wall has collapsed over the bevel. The in-line pressure resulting from a quick firm squeeze on the bulb is often all that is needed to clear the bevel so that the flow may resume.

11. Do you detect air in the tubing? Air not only slows the flow but also creates a potential embolic hazard. Ways by which you can rid air from the tubing include:

   a. Beginning directly below the lowest level of air in the tubing "thump," proceeding upward until the air escapes out of the tubing and is displaced above the solution (Figure 3-15).

   b. Twisting the tubing (beginning again below the level of air in the tubing) around a pen, scissors or other object will also displace the air out of the tubing (Figure 3-16).

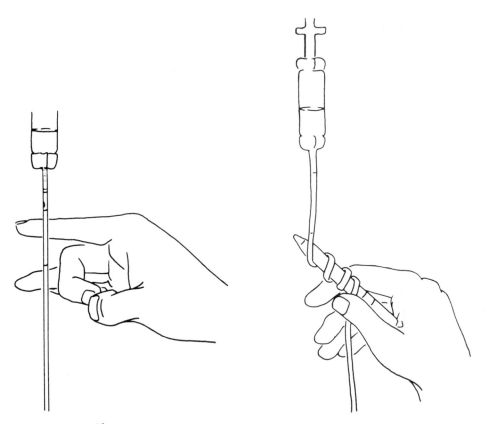

Figure 3-15   Figure 3-16

c. If the air is near the insertion site, if possible slow the flow; quickly wipe the circular indentations on the adaptor bulb with an antiseptic sponge; insert a sterile 25-gauge needle into the bulb; open the flow adaptor clamp—air will escape through the hub of the 25-gauge needle as the fluid continues into the vein. Once the air has escaped, remove the 25-gauge needle, and the site on the bulb is self-sealing; then regulate the flow rate (Figure 3-17).

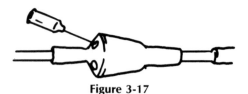

Figure 3-17

d. If there is a large quantity of air and/or if it is already very low in the tubing at the insertion site and there is no rubber bulb on the particular infusion set-up, then it becomes necessary to *disconnect* the tubing from the needle or catheter, permitting fluid and air to pass into a receptacle (e.g., emesis, basin, wastecan, etc.) momentarily until the line is cleared of air. However, extreme caution must be used to maintain sterility of the tubing and the needle hub and to prevent dislodging the needle from the vein (Figure 3-18).

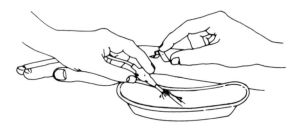

Figure 3-18

12. When measures fail to regulate the IV, it may be necessary to irrigate the site.
    a. Fill 1-ml tuberculin syringe with a small gauge needle, with sterile isotonic solution or withdraw a ml of the solution the patient is receiving from the rubber bulb. (This syringe will create more force and require the use of less solution than a larger barrel syringe.) Pinch the tubing proximal to the bulb, so that all the fluid forced into the line from the syringe is directed toward the insertion site (Figure 3-19).
    b. When there is no rubber bulb, turn off the flow rate; disconnect the tubing from the needle or catheter. With no needle on the syringe, connect the tuberculin syringe and irrigate. Remove syringe, reconnect line and turn on flow-rate clamp (note Figure 3-20).

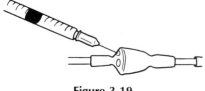

Figure 3-19

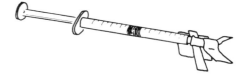

Figure 3-20

If the IV runs dry into the tubing, do not disconnect it if at all possible. If the IV runs dry and air enters the tubing, here is what to do especially if there is a stopcock in place:

1. Either pinch the tubing below the point where there is still fluid or turn the extension tubing stopcock to the central "off" position.
2. Wrap the tubing around and around your finger, forcing the air out of the tubing, up toward the drip chamber.
3. Once the air is completely out of the tubing, release the tubing wrapped around your finger.
4. Unpinch the tubing or return the stopcock to the proper position and adjust the flow rate. The IV line is then free of air.

This method is used to prevent having to disconnect the tubing to run the air out, which would increase the chance of contamination.

OTHER PEARLS FOR INTRAVENOUS THERAPY
Pearl (25) Discontinuing an IV

1. Turn off the flow rate.
2. Remove all tape and restraints.
3. Withdraw the needle or catheter slowly and smoothly in a straight line.
4. Apply pressure at the site (with use of a four-by-four gauze sponge folded in half), for 45 to 60 seconds.
5. Observe the site to determine if the sponge should be taped over the site or discarded. Sometimes a small amount of antimicrobial ointment is applied or a Band-Aid is needed.
6. Observe the needle and catheter tip to note any breaks.
7. It may be helpful to use adhesive remover when removing the tape.

Pearl (26) The Care of Patients Receiving IV Therapy

To facilitate the regulating of the infusion and maintaining accurate intake, place a strip of tape along the side of the solution bag and mark off the amount needed per hourly interval. This can be done more easily prior to hanging the solution container, usually at the same time the patient's name and solution identification tag are placed on the solution.

When hanging a new bottle, identify time, date, rate of infusion and who is hanging the solution (note Figure 3-21). When hanging several bags to infuse into one site through a stopcock, label the tubing near the stopcock to quickly identify each separate line (Figure 3-22). These labels may be color-coded.

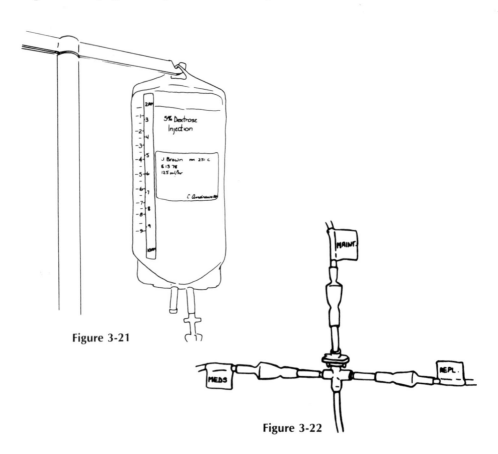

Figure 3-21

Figure 3-22

Pearl (27) Failure to Communicate—A Flaw in IV Therapy

Communicate to the staff caring for the patient the specific details regarding this patient's fluid needs. It is helpful to list the fluids to be infused, rate, and time one needs to hang the new solution bag. This can be placed on individual medication or treatment cards, on the nursing Kardex, and on the worksheet. This information should be shared in shift reports. Take note of infusion set-up when on nursing rounds.

Pearl (28) Become Familiar with the Specific Equipment

For instance, when using a Buritrol, Solu-set, Volutrol, etc., to regulate for a continuous flow at a slow KVO (keep vein open) rate, with some sets you simply clamp off the air filter and regulate flow. With other sets the air filter must remain open.

Pearl (29) IV Tray

It is much easier for the staff to keep all of the usual needed supplies for infusion assembled on a large tray or on a cart near the nurse's station. It should be metal or plastic for easy cleaning. Save small cardboard boxes (like those in which the alcohol wipes and gauze sponges are supplied) to keep the tray or infusion cart orderly.

Pearl (30) Label the IV Tubing

When multiple IV solutions are being infused intermittently through a stop-cock, it is very helpful to label the *tubing* near the stopcock rather than the IV bag or the tubing near the bag. This way the nurse does not have to trace all of the tubing to find the solution that she needs.

Also helpful is the use of color-coded tape: one color for each solution, marked on the bag and on the tubing near the stopcock.

Pearl (31) Cotton Swabs Useful in IV Care

Cotton swabs are smaller than four-by-fours or even two-by-twos. If used sterilely in IV care, they can allow the nurse to clean more thoroughly the hub of the IV needle and any part of an intravenous catheter that is exposed.
1. Open the swabs sterilely.
2. Saturate one swab with Betadine and keep the other one dry.
3. Clean the IV site with solution, then dry with the dry swab. Follow this with Betadine ointment and a dry sterile dressing, and IV care is done.

Helping promote adequate nutrition and hydration in the patient often requires a team effort. In addition to the nursing staff, many of the Pearls were shared with us by the fine staff in our dietary department, with Ms. Ruby Puckett as department head.

PEARLS FOR PATIENTS RECEIVING GASTRIC TUBE FEEDINGS
Pearl (32) Relieving Thirst

A person who is receiving gastrostomy feedings should not experience thirst. Feedings usually have sufficient amounts of fluids so that extra fluids are seldom needed. Should thirst occur, additional fluids may be necessary. But, as with any patient, it is best to consult with the dietitian when possible before offering fluids or foods.

Pearl (33) Preventing Constipation

Constipation may occur due to the lack of fiber in the diet. Often prune juice, as an extra fluid, and Karo syrup are added.

Pearl (34) Feedings for the Traveler

Vary the feedings by using Instant Breakfast and other such commercial products for ease in caring for the patient who is traveling.

Pearl (35) Whip Up a Batch of D₅W for a Feeding

If the doctor has ordered D₅W to follow a tube feeding, it will probably be quicker and easier to make your own than to wait for the pharmacy to send it. Also it will be cheaper than using IV fluid for a gastric feeding. A common restaurant size packet of sugar weighs 5 grams. Simply dissolve one packet of sugar in 100 cc of water. *Voila!* D₅W! (Only good for feeding, of course, *not for IV administration.*)

HELPING THE BLIND OR VISUALLY IMPAIRED PATIENT WITH MEALS

Pearl (36) Assistance at the Bedside

The nurse should have someone available to assist the blind patient at mealtimes when his tray arrives.

Pearl (37) Dishes with Rims

Use dishes that have sides or rims for helping blind patients feed themselves.

Pearl (38) Contrast with Color of Dishes

For the nearly blind or visually impaired patient, use dark-colored dishes. This aids in providing a visual contrast with the lighter-colored foods.

Pearl (39) Familiar Place

Always place foods in the same position on the tray and plate.

Pearl (40) Patience and Pace

Whether teaching the patient, orienting him to his environment or familiarizing him with certain routines, remember to adapt the intervention to compensate for the visual loss. Also give the patient time to assimilate the information which is given.

Pearl (41) The Food Tray Becomes a Clock

To encourage self-feeding for the patient who has a visual impairment because of bandages or physical problems, it is helpful to orient him to the *location* of the food on his tray by relating the plate to a clock. (In Figure 3-23, the milk is at 1 o'clock, the salad is at 11 o'clock, etc.)

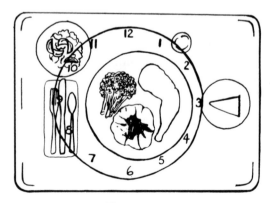

Figure 3-23

DIFFICULTY IN EATING
Pearl (42) Inverting the Straw

Dip the end of a straw in the liquid the patient is to consume. Then invert the straw end, placing the wet end of the straw in the patient's mouth. This is particularly helpful for the patient who has been NPO (nothing by mouth) and finds he has difficulty sipping through the straw with a dry mouth. The flavor of the liquid on the straw (broth, juice, etc.) also aids in stimulating his appetite.

Pearl (43) An Improvised Feeder

For patients who are alert enough to drink but have difficulty bringing liquids up through a straw or drinking with a cup or opening their mouths, and for the patient who has difficulty moving fluids from the front to the back of his mouth, try this: Attach three to four inches of rubber tubing to a 60 cc catheter tip syringe. Draw fluid up through the tubing, then place the end of the tubing in the patient's mouth in the position that is easiest for him to manage. Using this method, you can control the placement, the amount and the rate of oral liquid feedings.

Pearl (44) Feeding the Patient Who Has Dysphagia

The patient should be sitting in a semi-Fowler's position when at all possible. Place a small pillow or bath blanket under the shoulders so that his head is slightly hyperextended (Figure 3-24). When the liquid is ready to be placed in the mouth by cup, spoon, breakfeeder or syringe, support the back of the patient's head in your free hand. Tilt his head forward to a slightly anterior position as he receives fluid (Figure 3-25). Then *gradually* permit the patient's head to rest back in the hyperextended position as he swallows. This helps prevent aspiration from too rapid intake. The nurse is more in control of the situation. This support from the nurse also helps to provide some feeling of security for the patient.

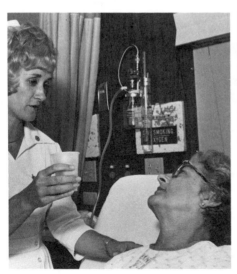

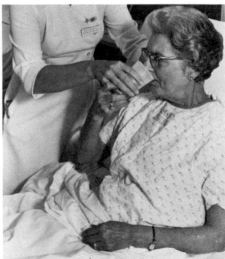

Figure 3-24   Figure 3-25

Pearl (45) Placing the Liquid Under the Tongue

When feeding the patient who has difficulty swallowing, place the liquid (by spoon, syringe, or whatever device) *under* rather than on top of the tongue. This eliminates too rapid ingestion and deters aspiration. After the fluid is placed under the tongue, assist the patient to slowly hyperextend his head. This facilitates the movement of the liquid toward the esophagus by gravity.

Pearl (46) Suction Ready—Forced Feedings

When such forced feeding methods must be used as alternatives to various intravenous therapies, one must use extreme caution to prevent untoward effects such as choking, coughing, etc. Oropharyngeal suction should be placed at the bedside. Turn suction to hi-vac and have the catheter attached.

STIMULATING THE APPETITE

Pearl (47) Forcing Fluids Through Rose Colored Straws

Johnny had surgery and now he will not drink his clear liquids? Try giving him a flexible colored straw. He may just ask for more.

Pearl (48) Use Favorite Color

If the patient is not eating well, it may help stimulate his appetite if his favorite color is used in a placemat or a decoration in his eating area.

Pearl (49) Avoid Negative Comments

Instruct staff, and set a role model yourself, in avoiding negative comments or gestures about the taste or consistency of the food. Such a negative attitude may affect the patient's acceptance of a dietary modification and/or even his appetite.

Pearl (50) Making Feedings More Acceptable

Supplemental feedings (such as Ensure) will appear more acceptable to the patient if it is served to him in a cup, possibly with a straw and sometimes over ice, rather than warm from a pop-top can (Figures 3-26 and 3-27).

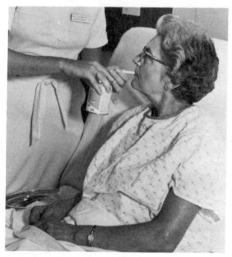

Figure 3-26

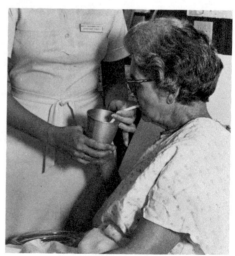

Figure 3-27

Pearl (51) Pleasant Mealtimes—Please!

While the mealtime may be a *convenient* time during the shift to assess some of your patient's daily needs or activities, *avoid* disrupting his mealtime. (Mealtime is *not the time* to check with the patient to assess if he has had a bowel movement.)

PLANNING THE INTAKE
Pearl (52) Consult with the Dietitian

When patients are on therapeutic diets such as with potassium, fluid, sodium, carbohydrate, and other restrictions, consult with the dietitian. Remember that managing the patient regarding this dietary restriction and proper nutrition often requires the expertise of the dietitian, an indispensible and valuable member of the health team.

Pearl (53) Assessing Fluid Needs

Initiate an assessment of the particular patient situation in collaboration with the dietitian when at all possible. Such an assessment should clarify:
1. What is the patient's preferences of liquids (i.e., apple juice versus orange juice, etc.)?
2. Will he need fluids to mix or accompany medications? If so, how much, at what times of the day?
3. What is the patient's activity level?
4. Is he febrile? Does he perspire profusely?
5. Should he receive more fluids on one shift than on others?

Pearl (54) Formulating a Plan

Once a plan has been formulated, it is essential that the staff, patient, and family are well informed about the plan. This may require:
1. Posting a fluid schedule at the bedside, such as the one illustrated in Figure 3-28, written on a four-by-six card: FR—total daily fluid intake allotted; K—kitchen (fluid that will be furnished and sent at the established times by the dietary department); the D, E, and N designate the fluid allotment which the nurses on the day, evening and night shifts will give to the patient.

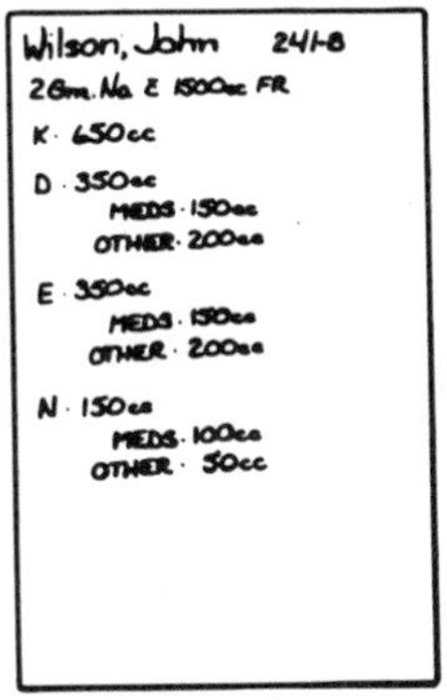

Figure 3-28

2.   Posting a note of the schedule in the Kardex and on the team leader worksheet as a reminder to inform nursing staff on each oncoming shift.

3.   Communicating with the dietary department and/or the physician should certain situations occur which might alter the patient's fluid intake needs, such as: the patient losing fluid by vomiting, perspiring due to fever, refusing to take certain fluids, or being NPO for certain diagnostic tests. *An accurate intake and output record is essential.* Often patients who have fluid restrictions or who are NPO will find much comfort in such palliative measures as good oral hygiene, mouth rinses, tart lemon drops, peppermints or other hard candies as the diet permits. Ice chips should not be used as a substitute because they add up eventually to increased intake and have not been found helpful in quenching thirst.

MEASURING THE INTAKE
Pearl (55) Measuring the Intake Accurately

Staff consistency in measurements helps to provide a more accurate measurement of the patient's oral intake.

A list of measurements for various receptacles (i.e., cup, juice glass, etc.) with capacities in milliliters for each should be easily accessible to the staff responsible for these intake records.

Three common places which are easily accessible are:
1.   Taped to the rack at each bedside which holds the intake-output flow sheet.
2.   Xeroxed on back of the flow sheets (with pictorial diagrams of the receptacles if the patient is assisting with measuring his own intake).
3.   By the lavatory in the patient's bathroom.

Pearl (56) Fluid Restrictions—How to Keep the Intake Accurate

Once the physician has ordered that the patient be limited to a particular intake of fluids, several steps must be taken to ensure that a sensible daily intake plan is implemented (see Pearl 54).

ALTERING LIFETIME DIETARY HABITS
Pearl (57) The Sweet Tooth

The geriatric patient often prefers foods with a high carbohydrate and sugar content. Some of the reasons for this are:
1.   Diet patterns which have been established over a lifetime.
2.   They are easier to masticate.
3.   The erroneous idea that sugar is a "quick energy" source. (This is not true unless the person is near starvation.)
4.   These foods are often less expensive than high protein foods.
Teach the patient that sugar harms:
1.   By leading to obesity due to the added caloric intake.
2.   When it takes the place of a well-balanced diet (i.e., a candy bar often may dampen the desire for more nourishing foods).
3.   Because it plays a role in the arteriosclerotic process, though the exact mechanism is not yet fully understood.

Pearl (58) Egg Beaters and Egg Substitutes

Many geriatric patients have long-established dietary patterns which include the use of eggs. Suggest that they limit the number of eggs per week and when possible use egg substitutes (such as Egg Beaters) which eliminate the high cholesterol intake. Bake with the whites of the eggs only—they have less cholesterol and fewer calories.

Elimination
Chapter four

In caring for patients, nurses have the opportunity and responsibility for:
1. Promoting proper elimination
2. Teaching safe and healthful habits of elimination
3. Accurately assessing the patient's elimination process
4. Identifying factors that can effect change in the elimination patterns for each individual

This chapter presents Pearls which you can apply in the daily care of your patients who have various elimination needs. *Some specific considerations include:*

Pearls for the patient with a colostomy
Pearls for dealing with the problem of incontinence and catheter management
Pearls for aiding the patient with altered bowel habits
Pearls for assessing and managing drainage (postop, gastric suction, etc.)

COLOSTOMY AND WOUND DRAINS
Pearl (1) Preop Assessment

If it is suspected or known preoperatively that a colostomy will be performed on the patient, it is crucial that 1) the physician (initially) and the nurse discuss this procedure with the patient. The preoperative care should include encouragement of the patient to share his feelings and questions. 2) When at all possible, the nurse should collaborate with the physician to assist him in determining the best site for the ostomy stoma prior to going into the operating room. This permits the patient to change positions (i.e., lying, sitting) to help determine the best stoma site, since, for example, a fold of fat or bony prominence may not be obvious when the patient is supine or on the OR table. Such factors often make it difficult postoperatively to keep a stoma appliance fitting securely to eliminate leakage. If your hospital is fortunate enough to have an enterostomal therapist, she can be a terrific source of help in coordinating this patient's care.

Pearl (2) Cleaning the Stoma Site

One of the problems which can be prevented or minimized is irritation to the skin from the drainage. Cleaning with soap and water on the skin about the stoma and applying the disposable stoma bag securely to prevent leakage are helpful.

Pearl (3) When to Change the Stoma Bag

Stoma bags should be changed only when absolutely necessary, as when they begin to loosen from the skin. Too frequent removal of the stoma bag irritates the skin.

Pearl (4) An Asepto for Flushing the Soiled Bag

If the bag becomes soiled, it can be flushed clear from the distal end of the bag by using an asepto syringe and solution.

Pearl (5) Using the Red Robinson

Another method of cleaning the bag is by cutting a small opening, approximately the size of a dime, in the portion of the stoma bag above the stoma. A small Red Robinson catheter can be slipped into this dime-size opening and the bag flushed clear with solution. Close the opening with tape.

Pearl (6) Karaya Rings

Karaya rings aid by adhering to the skin and keeping the bag in place. These rings also aid in the healing process. Frequently they are a part of the stoma bag.

Pearl (7) Applying Karaya Rings

When applying the karaya ring, hold it in your hands a moment to warm the karaya. This makes it more pliable to mold it to a shape to better fit the stoma.

Immediately before applying the karaya ring, quickly moisten it and apply from below the stoma in an upward direction over the stoma. Apply pressure to the ring and hold it a few moments as it dries and adheres to the skin.

Pearl (8) Artificial Stimulation

Some patients will require irrigations and others will not. If irrigation is necessary at any time, here are a few practices which we have found helpful.
1. Begin irrigations at the time of day that the patient will find most suitable to his life style at home.
2. Often an *irrigating cone* is preferred rather than the catheter. Why? It is less likely to perforate the intestine or traumatize the stomal tissues, it provides for easier insertion and it helps prevent backflow as you irrigate.
3. Use of an irrigating plastic bag (such as the Stoma Irrigator Drain by Hollister, Inc.) can be used. Allow the bag to drain between the patient's legs as he sits on the toilet.
4. Once the irrigation is completed, it is *not necessary for the patient to remain on the toilet* while he waits 30 to 60 minutes for the return of the solution. The distal end of the irrigating bag can be clamped or folded and tied with a rubber band as the patient shaves, applies makeup, reads, etc.
5. Use lukewarm tap water for irrigation; rid the tubing of air by flushing the fluid

through the tubing before beginning the irrigation. Keep the lower end of the enema can or bag no higher than the patient's shoulder level (when he is sitting on the toilet) to irrigate; have the patient massage his abdomen as the fluid is being instilled.

All these measures help prevent cramps and promote greater retention of the irrigating solution.

Pearl (9) Rectal Tenderness

Sometimes it is helpful to have the patient sit in a chair on a moderately inflated ring facing the toilet as he performs his colostomy care (for example, those patients who have perineal or rectal discomfort or tenderness from hemorrhoids or abdominal perineal resection, etc.).

Pearl (10) Eliminating Unpleasant Odor

Various measures can be used to try to eliminate odors. Some measures include:

1. Taking certain medication by mouth such as charcoal, chlorophyll, bismuth subcarbonate, etc. Consult with your doctor before taking any medications.
2. Maintaining cleanliness about the stoma site and of a soiled bag.
3. Eliminating certain gas-forming foods such as cabbage, beer, turnips, etc. However, this will vary with the individual.
4. Preventing possible blockage of the stoma passage, particularly if it is quite small. Corn-on-the-cob, popcorn, nuts, and other small items should be chewed thoroughly. Do not frighten your patient about possible blockage because with normal chewing this blockage is most uncommon.
5. Use room deodorizers in the bathroom.
6. Place an asprin or a safe deodorant in the stoma bag or use odor-proof plastic pouches (consult with the doctor and/or enterostomal therapist for additional measures).

Pearl (11) Expelling Flatus

Place two or three pinpricks in the superior portion of the stoma bag. This prevents back-up pressure which can cause cramping, as the flatus produces a ballooning of the stoma bag. The alert patient who is independent in caring for his colostomy may eliminate these pinpricks to avoid embarrassing odor as the gas escapes. He can be instructed to periodically open the distal end of the stoma bag in the bathroom to prevent the gas from accumulating too much in the bag.

Pearl (12) For Additional Assistance in Preventing Soiling of Clothes

In addition to the stoma bags, there are many types of materials designed to cover the stoma and prevent soiling of the clothes.

You, as well as the patient, will find that the enterostomal therapist, literature about colostomy care, and another person who has had a colostomy for some time will be very helpful resources.

Pearl (13) The Spouse and Patient's Adjustment

Include the family (and particularly the spouse) when at all possible in the teaching of the ostomy patient. Have them in on the teaching at an early stage. This is essential if they are going to recognize the patient's progress (for instance decrease in the size of the stoma).

Encourage the patient and his spouse to discuss their feelings, fears and expectations. No spouse should have to endure the psychological trauma caused by having the initial introduction to the spouse's change in body image (colostomy) alone, without the support of the health team, at home.

Pearl (14) Crotchless Panties

For sexual activity for women with ostomy pouches, suggest the use of crotchless panties which control gravity pull on the pouch and hide the contents.

Pearl (15) Emptying the Ostomy Pouch

To keep hands clean when emptying the colostomy pouch, turn back the end of the pouch to make a cuff, this also keeps the end of the pouch clean and dry.

Pearl (16) Formula for Karaya Paste

When out of karaya paste, mix karaya powder and glycerin until the consistency desired is reached.

Pearl (17) Uses of Stomahesive (by Swibb Co.)

1.   Stomahesive can be used on stumps to protect tender areas from the prostheses.

2.   It can be used for bandaging, to protect skin from tape burns. Place a piece of stomahesive where the tape normally falls. The tape can be put on or taken off stomahesive many times before stomahesive needs changing.

3.   It can be used for a reddened sacrum. Apply a piece of stomahesive over the area and leave it in place two days. This relieves pressure and promotes healing where there are draining wounds, penroses, or a pouch with ostomy bags. It also saves nursing time, expense and it keeps the patient dry. With draining wounds one can not obtain the correct size pouch. Use sandwich bags (Ziploc are odor-proof) and cement them to stomahesive.

USES OF BABY BOTTLE NIPPLES
Pearl (18) Draining the Ostomy Pouch

To attach the ostomy pouch to a straight drain:
1.   Cut a hole in the top of the nipple.
2.   Twist the end of the ostomy bag and put it through the hole in the nipple.
3.   Stick the end of the tube up through the end of the pouch and hole in nipple.

Pearl (19) On the End of Enema Tube

In doing a colostomy irrigation the nipple acts as a dam to keep water in.

For the patient who can not retain an enema, put the nipple in the rectum and hold it tightly in place.

Pearl (20) Bottle Nipples Eliminate Messy Drainage

Save time, provide continuous drainage, promote asepsis and eliminate those messy drainage systems by applying the bottle nipple method, as illustrated in

Figures 4-1 and 4-2. This improvized method can be used for all types of wound drains, such as when using stoma bags, when irrigating wounds, and for the patient with drainage fistulas.

1. Cut the top off the rubber bottle nipple.
2. Push the distal end of the drainage bag through the nipple opening (using bandage scissors or forceps, as necessary).
3. Then pull the distal end of the bag until two to four inches of the bag is through the nipple.
4. Connect the drainage tubing through the lower opening of the bag up into the distal end of the nipple (Figure 4-1). (The tubing is already connected to a drainage bag. We use the same type of closed-drainage system which is used in urinary drainage "set-ups.")
5. Pull the nipple downward over the end of the drainage tube (Figure 4-2).

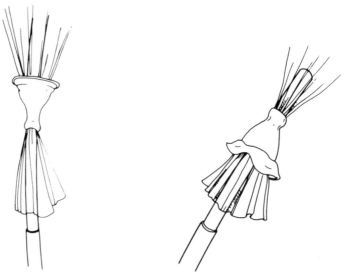

Figure 4-1   Figure 4-2

Pearl (21) Ostomy Pouch for Drainage

To put the ostomy pouch over the tube or area that is draining profusely:

1. Cut a hole in the pouch as usual.
2. Slit the backing on the pouch into two pieces, *but leave it in place.*
3. Wash and dry skin, then pull the tube through the hole in the pouch.
4. Take the top half of the backing off the pouch and stick it in place.
5. Put a four-by-four (gauze sponge) into the pouch and stuff it around the base of the tubes to catch drainage.
6. Take the remaining half of the backing off the pouch and apply it quickly.

Pearl (22) Low-Vac Suction for Copious Drainage

For ostomies or wounds with large amounts of drainage, hook the bedside drainage tubing to low-vac wall suction.

Pearl (23) Prone Position? Protect Stoma

For patients with ostomies who must be prone, place a soft foam ring under the abdomen around the stoma and pouch.

Pearl (24) Bottle Nipple for G-Tube

To prevent the gastrostomy (G-tube) tube from slipping from the incision site, insert the distal (external) end of the G-tube through a bottle nipple. (The very tip of the nipple has been cut away.) The nipple is pulled snugly against the skin so that the remaining tip of the nipple occludes the space about the G-tube.

Pearl (25) Postop Drainage

An important priority for intervening during the early postoperative period is assessing for drainage from the incision. Some points to consider in noting and early detection of drainage include the following:

1. Circle the drainage noted on dressing. It provides a visual estimate of the amount of drainage to report or record as necessary (e.g., "Dressing has a serosanguineous drainage spot the size of a half-dollar").

2. If the patient is lying supine, checking the dressing is not enough. Place hands along sides of the patient and underneath his back. Remember that drainage flows easily by gravity, thus much more drainage may exist than the external dressing reveals. This drainage is less apparent, the more bulky the dressing (e.g., with the patient following a mastectomy or a radical neck dissection).

3. While caring for the patient who has oral or throat surgery (e.g., thyroidectomy, tonsillectomy) the nurse should be alert to frequent swallowing by the patient as a clue to possible bleeding.

NASOGASTRIC DRAINAGE

Should the nasogastric tube, which is connected to intermittent suction, fail to function adequately, consider using the following Pearls.

Pearl (26) Position Change

Change the patient's position from side to side at intervals.

Pearl (27) Adjust the Bed

Elevate or lower the head of the bed.

Pearl (28) Irrigate the Catheter

Irrigating the catheter can be done by inserting saline and aspirating for the return. In some cases (such as immediately following gastrointestinal surgery) fluid cannot be used. In such cases, irrigate with one to two ounces of air and immediately connect the catheter to the suction apparatus.

Pearl (29) Rotate the Catheter

Gently rotate the catheter one full turn. This often prevents discomfort which occurs due to constant pressure of the catheter in one area of the throat.

Pearl (30) Is the Gastric Tube in the Stomach?

Each time before any solution, feeding or irrigant is inserted via the nasogastric tube into the stomach, it is essential to check if the tube is in the stomach. Otherwise the feeding can be aspirated into the lungs, causing severe complications.

While one may read in different sources a variety of ways to check for the catheter placement, there is *one* preferred way!

1. *Preferred way*
   a. Place the bell of the stethoscope on the abdomen.
   b. Insert a small amount of air with a syringe through the tube, while listening for bowel sounds from this air being inserted. (If the stethoscope is on the stomach, you *will* hear the sound as the air enters.)
2. *Disadvantages of the other methods*
   a. Aspirating for gastric contents. If aspirate returns, this may indicate correct tube placement. The problems are: if a fistula exists—and *if* no aspirate returns—then what? For the patient who has been NPO for a period of time, there may well be no gastric contents to aspirate.
   b. Placing the external end of the catheter into a cup of water. If it does not bubble it is not in the lungs. This is probably a reasonable assumption, but does it necessarily indicate the catheter is then in the stomach? *NO.* The catheter could be lying right below the uvula in the oropharynx or anywhere in the oronasal passage. Should this be the case and the feeding is inserted, the fluid could readily push the catheter into the trachea, thus entering the lungs.

Pearl (31) A Step Further Than the Flash or Click

It is simply not enough to glance at the suction machine to note if the light flashes on and off or if the suction machine clicks intermittently. This is only one step in determining if the patient is receiving adequate intermittent gastric suctioning. Here is a handy questionnaire for better assessment:
1. Is the patient vomiting while connected to suction?
2. Is there adequate drainage in the receptacle?
3. Is the abdomen distended?
4. When you disconnect tubing from the catheter, will the machine suction water? (Early checking of this step can prevent untoward problems.)

Place the tip of the tubing in a cup containing 10 to 15 cc of water to note if the water is suctioned from the cup. *Do not forget* to include this amount on the output sheet.

Here are a few Pearls which you may find helpful in winning the patient's cooperation for an easier insertion of the nasogastric tube.

Pearl (32) High Fowler's

The patient should be sitting in an upright position with a pillow behind his head to produce a slight forward flexion. This helps prevent accidentally inserting the catheter into the trachea.

Pearl (33) Protector

Place a Chux (or other protective covering) across the patient's chest and across his lap to prevent possible soiling of the linens from vomitus or drainage, etc.

Pearl (34) Diversion

After explanations of the procedure to the patient, give him something to do to divert his attention to some extent (e.g., ask him to hold the emesis basin so that the end of the catheter can rest in it as you insert the tube).

Pearl (35) Another Basin—Please

With some patients it is helpful to substitute another basin instead of the emesis basin. This is particularly true when the very sight of an emesis basin makes the patient gag or become nauseated.

Pearl (36) Firm Insistence

When inserting the catheter through the nares, proceed slowly following the *floor* of the passage. Once through the area of the turbinates, you will feel almost no resistance. At that point, pause a moment, and then calmly, firmly, and slowly give further instruction, asking him to "swallow, swallow, swallow," as you more rapidly proceed with the insertion of the catheter through the pharynx, esophagus, and into the stomach. By responding to this simple instruction, the patient tends to have less time for gagging.

Pearl (37) Hazard of Water

While taking sips of water as the tube is being inserted may make swallowing easier, it is not recommended. Why? a) The patient may spill the water on himself unless you have another staff person to hold the cup of water; b) the sips of water may produce vomiting; c) the patient is often NPO; and d) due to his often high stress level, there is always the potential for choking and aspirating the water into the trachea.

Pearl (38) How to Measure the Length of the Catheter to Be Inserted

Measure the catheter from tip of nose to the earlobe to the xiphoid process. Place the tape one to one and a half inches onto the catheter beyond this measurement. Consequently, the catheter should be in the stomach and the taped portion of the catheter should be at the immediate external nasal orifice.

While markings are usually placed by the manufacturer on the tubing at various distances, the distance to each individual's stomach varies. The tape serves as a reminder to *stop the catheter insertion* at that point before entering the nares.

Pearl (39) Tee the Tube

When the patient with a nasogastric tube can ambulate without having the tube connected to suction, several methods can be used to clamp the tube.

We found the use of golf tees, which come in various sizes, helpful. The tee is used to plug the external end of the tube. Thus, there is no leakage and no wear and tear of the tube.

BLADDER AND BOWEL ELIMINATION
Pearl (40) Taping the Foley Securely and Comfortably

There is a handy way to tape Foley catheters to provide a maximum amount of comfort and movement without pulling. You need:
1. Six-inch piece of two-inch adhesive tape
2. Six-inch piece of one-inch adhesive tape
3. Two-by-two gauze square *or* 2 cotton-tipped applicators
4. Bottle of benzoin
5. Rubber band
6. Safety pin

First cleanse the thigh or abdominal well. Then apply benzoin liberally, with gauze or applicators. When the benzoin becomes tacky, apply the two-inch adhesive tape to the skin. Make a one-inch tab in the middle of the one-inch adhesive tape, then tape it to the two-inch tape.

Take a rubber band, wrap it around the portion of the catheter to be secured, and slip it through itself. Fix it with a safety pin to the one-inch tape tab and the catheter is secure (note Figure 4-3). Figure 4-4 depicts an alternate method.

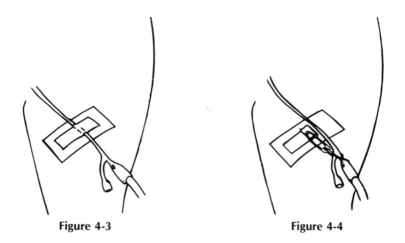

Figure 4-3   Figure 4-4

Pearl (41) The Sex Denotes Where to Tape the Catheter

Prior to taping the Foley catheter, shave the excess hair at the site where the tape is to be placed. In *women* tape the catheter to the inner aspect of the thigh (Figure 4-5). In *men* tape the catheter on the *lower* abdomen. This *prevents* the alteration in the normal direction of urine flow and the potential for fistula formation (Figure 4-6).

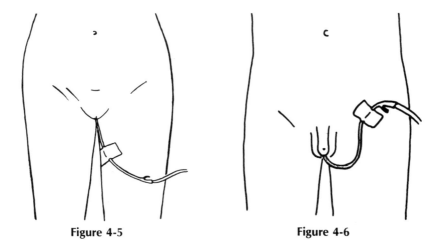

Figure 4-5   Figure 4-6

Pearl (42) Discontinuing the Foley Catheter

Prior to the removal of the Foley, it is important to note the size of the balloon of that particular Foley. This can be found printed on the external part of the catheter. To eliminate unnecessary trips to seek this information, record the size of the balloon as well as the size of the catheter at the time of insertion on the nurse's notes and the patient's care plan Kardex. If inserted in the operating room or postanesthesia recovery, record the information on the appropriate sheets for these areas. This will guide you in selecting the correct syringe size for deflating the balloon as you assemble the equipment.

Following are additional Pearls to consider in safely deflating a catheter.

Pearl (43) No Cutting the Catheter

Avoid cutting the catheter to allow deflation of the balloon. Why? Occasionally, the balloon may not deflate completely for various reasons, such as adherence of the balloon to clots or calculi formation. If the catheter is withdrawn without deflation, it can traumatize the bladder, and urethra.

Pearl (44) Avoid Overinflation

Teach the staff to avoid overinflation of the balloon. Different catheters have different size balloons, so select the correct size in advance, and instill the correct amount of fluid in the balloon.

Pearl (45) No Syringe Available

Occasionally, as in a home situation, the syringe is not available because of expense, etc. One can improvise safely by deflating the balloon with the stick end of an applicator, providing a receptacle to collect the return for measurement is available to assess if all the fluid is removed from the balloon.

Pearl (46) Use Sterile Thumb Forceps
Urinary Catheterization Procedure

Clean the meatus using a sterile thumb forcep prior to the insertion of the catheter into the meatus. This provides much greater control in maintaining sterility.

Pearl (47) The External Catheter

Urinary incontinence creates such problems for the patient as excoriated skin, discomfort, odoriferous surroundings and often much embarrassment.

The nurse is confronted with the task of selecting an appropriate means of helping the patient control this problem. One of the most successful measures when caring for the male patient is the use of the external catheter. When this is correctly applied and a careful hygienic regimen is followed, the problems associated with urinary incontinence are greatly decreased and often alleviated (note Figure 4-7).

A supply of these catheters can be made by the staff in advance. The items needed in constructing the condom catheter are the following:
1. 5 cm length of Tygon (firm plastic) tubing, 1 cm in diameter.
2. Plastic stopper 1 cm in length which will fit snugly into the Tygon tubing.
3. 5 cm length of velcro or Elastoplast strip (approximately 2.5 to 3 cm in width).
4. Condom.

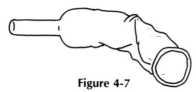

Figure 4-7

Pearl (48) How to Apply the External Catheter

Clean the penis with soap and water and dry thoroughly, making certain the foreskin is returned to the normal position over the glans before applying the external catheter (otherwise local circulatory impairment can occur due to swelling from the constricting foreskin).

Unroll the condom, pulling it upward and over the penis, and secure it with the strip of Elastoplast or velcro by wrapping it around the condom once, avoiding the skin. Then attach the condom catheter to the external drainage receptacle (see Figure 4-8).

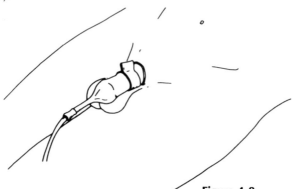

Figure 4-8

Pearl (49) Keeping the External Catheter Patent

Inspect the catheter soon after applying and then several times each shift in order to detect any twisting of the condom. Twisting of the condom occurs often in the restless patient who is frequently changing positions. A twisted external catheter obstructs urine output. Also note any edema of the glans penis. This can be eliminated by loosening the strip of velcro or Elastoplast. In addition to looking for any signs of obstruction or irritation, careful cleaning of the penis, external catheter changes periodically, usually twice a day, and application of an antibacterial ointment when necessary are important.

Pearl (50) Propped Urinal

When a urinal must be propped between the patient's legs in order to catch the urine, which is often the case for the bedridden patient who is incontinent and has an excoriated penile area, place a Chux under the urinal to prevent wetting the linen and the patient.

By the way, this can only be used in the patient who is *not* restless or who is alert and can change or ask for a change in the urinal as he changes positions in the bed.

Pearl (51) Leg Urinals

Use a leg urinal for those patients who are incontinent and have an indwelling or external catheter. This permits the patient to ambulate with greater ease than if he had to carry a large drainage bag (Figure 4-9).

To care for the leg urinals, wash with soap and water and rinse with a mild antiseptic solution and air-dry thoroughly. The patient who has the rubber leg urinals for long-term use needs at least two urinals. This will permit him to wear one while the other is drying.

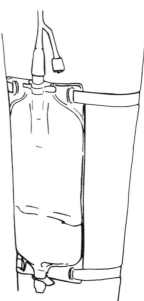

Figure 4-9

Pearl (52) Urinary Incontinence—Care of the Woman

There are various styles and sizes of plastic lined panties which can be used by the woman with urinary incontinence. These can be purchased at a surgical supply store and some neighborhood pharmacies.

The nurse will find, however, that on many occasions she must improvize. Some improvisions follow:

1.   Enclosing the sides and bottom of the superabsorbent sanitary napkin with a piece of plastic (e.g., cut from a plastic-lined Chux) securing the edges with tape. The ends of the napkins are attached to the sanitary belt. The patient can change these pads herself.

2.   Fashioning two triangles by cutting two plastic Chux, lined lightly with absorbent material. The triangles are pinned at the waist and overlapped at the perineum where they are then pinned. Additional padding can be provided at the perineum by enclosing a heavy ABD pad such as a heavy drainage pack. The amount of padding will vary to meet the individual patient's needs. The absorbent pads can be changed by unpinning the Chux at the perineum (note Figure 4-10).

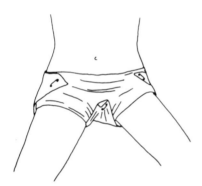

Figure 4-10

Pearl (53) Eliminating the Nighttime Bathroom Trek

For patients who have problems ambulating or become disoriented at night and who need to use the bathroom, keep the urinal, bedside commode, or bedpan at the bedside. This helps to prevent falls, etc.

Pearl (54) The Bedpan Is Not Enough

The patient asks to use the bedpan. You should provide him with a call light, a roll of toilet tissue, a Chux to protect the bed linen, a Chux to cover the bedpan.

Such provisions aid by eliminating unnecessary trips to the bedside, preventing embarrassment, and providing reassurance that help can be summoned as needed.

Pearl (55) Bedpans Don't *Have* to Be Cold

Warm the bedpan by holding it under warm water. When you put the patient on it, not only will you have a grateful patient, but you will decrease the difficulty of using the bedpan, perhaps avoiding constipation or urinary retention.

Pearl (56) Difficulty Voiding

For women having difficulty voiding, put ammonia or oil of wintergreen on cotton and put this in the bedpan. It helps stimulate voiding.

Pearl (57) Early Voiding

Encourage the patient to void prior to a preop medication, pelvic exam, enema and other procedures. Why?
1. This helps decrease unnecessary restlessness when he is anxious over the impending procedure by eliminating a full bladder.
2. This allows the patient to rest quietly for maximum effects from the medication without having to be disturbed to use the urinal or bedpan.
3. This allows better examination and palpation of the pelvic organs.
4. This permits greater retention of the enema solution.

Pearl (58) Ready to Measure the Output?

Measurement of the output is made simple by keeping a graduated metal or plastic receptacle in the patient's bathroom. This avoids unnecessary delays leading to inadvertent spilling or discarding of the specimen.

Pearl (59) The Elderly Patient's Elimination Regimen

One of the most annoying problems faced by the hospitalized geriatric is his loss of control in managing his long-established routine for effective elimination. You can help prevent this problem by assessing what his usual routine is. (Is it a glass of warm water, hot coffee, or glass of juice before breakfast; a glass of prune juice at bedtime, or two tablespoons of milk of magnesia or other laxatives every other day.) When his past routine involves the use of a medication, consult with the physician regarding an order.

Psychosocial

Chapter five

Why nursing? Ask this question of a hundred nursing colleagues and you will receive a variety of responses. However, it has been our experience that a central theme tends to prevail: "I wanted to care for people," "I enjoy working with people," etc. Being "people oriented" certainly is important in nursing.

Experiencing a sense of satisfaction and happiness from helping others is but one of the *many* rewards inherent in being a nurse.

For instance, as you intervene in helping the patient deal with his psychosocial needs, an awareness of your own feelings and a better understanding of yourself develops.

This skill of effectively relating to others requires practice; self-awareness and a genuine concern for others.

Effective communication is a vital part of psychotherapeutic nursing intervention. Poor communication creates a level of stress which can impair the nurse-patient relationship and even potentially hinder the patient's progress in coping with his psychosocial needs and problems.

The nurse must recognize that the degree of control which the patient maintains and perceives he maintains as he deals with such stress as hospitalization, severity of illness, and separation from the family significantly influences the nurse-patient interaction.

In this chapter you will find:
1. Pearls for communicating with patients and family
2. Pearls for helping the patient cope with his problems
3. Pearls for caring for the patient with special limitations
4. Pearls which help promote independence and a sense of being in control

To start at the beginning, here are 10 Pearls that deal with interactions with the hospitalized child. Following them we will look at the other end of the life cycle with Pearls that concern interactions with the hospitalized geriatric patient.

THE PEDIATRIC PATIENT

Pearl (1) Stroking the Baby

Young infants have no way to understand that the treatments they receive, though painful, are therapeutic. That is why our nurses in the neonatal intensive care unit purposely stroke the infant after painful procedures. The warmth of human contact helps to reassure the crying baby.

Pearl (2) A Message to Parents

When parents can participate in even a small way in the care of their infant, this should be encouraged to strengthen parent-child interaction. One measure which we use to increase infant-bonding is to:

Tape a note to the crib, displaying the infant's footprint by his name, with a message to the parents such as the following:

1. "Dear Mom and Dad, please rub my back," signed Joey.
2. "Dear Parents, you may feed me now," signed Janie. These simple messages make the visits more meaningful.

Pearl (3) A Sneak-Preview

Provide an orientation booklet for the child who is being admitted to the hospital. This is particularly meaningful when the hospitalization is to be a new experience for the child.

Suggestions in preparing and using the booklet:

1. Make it personal.
   a. For instance, give it a title: *My First Hospital Visit.*
   b. Leave a space for the child to write his own name, e.g., this book belongs to *Joey Smith.*
   c. Use personal pronouns such as "you" rather than "the child."
   d. Provide an envelope inside the cover for him to place small memorabilia (e.g., hospital identification bracelet, get-well cards, etc.).
2. Present in a simple story form, using sketches for him to color, which reinforce the orientation story.
3. Use a positive approach (the Do's versus Don'ts).
4. This can be distributed at the clinics, at the local physicians' offices, at the admissions office, or by the nursing staff on the pediatric units if orientation visits are provided.
5. Encourage the parents and child to read through the book together. Suggest to the parents that they may wish to encourage their child to share his thoughts about the pictures he is coloring.
6. If the child elects to bring the book to the hospital, the staff should continue assisting him in using his personal booklet throughout the hospital stay.

Such a booklet aids by providing the parents with an active role in better preparing their child for his new experience. It also helps allay the child's apprehension about his unknown (new) venture.

Pearl (4) Clarifying Terms with Children

Listen to and encourage feedback from children when they are given explanations. Too often the simple explanation is misunderstood by the child because of a misinterpretation of the use of terms (e.g., use of "die" and "dye").

Two methods of assessing if the child understands the use of certain terms are to:

1. Follow up the explanation with a discussion in which the youngster can ask questions and will feel free to give his opinions and expectations.
2. Use unstructured play (e.g., having the child draw a picture and tell you what he thinks you have told him; using hand puppets with him to encourage his "acting out"; and story telling).

Pearl (5) A Cast with Character

Wearing a cast is certainly no fun for the patient. But we have found that "dressing up" the cast makes it more tolerable or acceptable to the patient, particularly the child or teenager. From materials on hand, you or the family can create your own easy design which would appeal to the particular individual. Such fancy casts include the tuxedo look, the favorite pet, the football, etc. This also seems to help the young patient to deal with communicating more positively with others. At the very least it helps divert that habitual question, "What happened to you?"

Pearl (6) Sneaker Casts

Spark up those ankle-length casts for the youngsters by coloring them as sneakers. For added diversion, assist or encourage them to design their own "sneakers."

Pearl (7) The Fun Soak

You can win the child's cooperation in soaking his extremity when needed by making it a time to play. (Examples: place small plastic objects or pebbles in the water for the child to reach in and then place them in a plastic container; or fill a squeeze bottle and place it in the basin and have him squeeze or step on the plastic bottle while it is underwater, by squirting the water out of the bottle. This takes time and makes bubbles, adding to the fun.)

Pearl (8) Pantomimes and Funny Faces

To promote exercise in children postoperatively win their cooperation by:

1. Giving explanations based on their level of understanding.
2. Having them first move body parts which do not hurt.
3. Creating pantomimes that permit them to move extremities and change positions. (Tell a story that requires them to act out the characters. The characters may need to pretend to run bases, ride a bike, reach and pull on the tower bell, blow the policeman's whistle, etc.)
4. Providing them with colorful balloons to blow (much more appealing to youngsters than the "blow-glove").
5. Giving them a container with a small amount of water and a straw to make bubbles by blowing through the straw. (The child should not be NPO for this

activity. He must also be alert and old enough to use a straw without sucking inward through it.)
6. Watching them make funny faces while looking in a mirror.

Pearl (9) Talking with the Adolescent

When talking with the adolescent, get the adolescent alone. Others, particularly other adolescents, cause much peer pressure. You will find the adolescent is much more open and honest when with only one adult.

Pearl (10) The Snapshots—Show and Tell

Snapshots can serve many useful purposes, particularly in the care of children. Snapshots can:
1. Portray a visual account of a child's growth and development.
2. Enhance the staff's awareness of the positive effects of therapy and of their efforts in providing patient care.
3. Decrease high-level stress in parents and their youngsters, who are anxious in beginning a new or long-term therapy program (e.g., dialysis, physical therapy).
4. Provide a means of sharing with friends the good news of becoming new parents.
   Situations in which we have found using snapshots helpful include:
1. Posting snapshot of the newborn in the infant's crib or bassinet shortly after the admission to newborn intensive care units (NICU).
2. Preparing a bulletin board of snapshots, which are often received weeks or even months later from the parents of the youngsters who have been discharged from the dialysis unit. This bulletin board is placed where new admissions and their parents can see it and share their comments with the staff. It is reassuring for them to see progress that has been made in such a therapy program with other children.
3. Providing a snapshot of that newborn for the proud parents to share with family and friends.

THE GERIATRIC PATIENT

Here is a string of Pearls that bring new ideas to the care of geriatric patients:

Pearl (11) The Good Ole Days

It is important to listen to the elderly patient reminisce, as you will often learn much about the patient that will be helpful as you prepare the care plan.

However, it is equally important to help the elderly patient focus some of his attention to the present and future. This can be done by using such aids as discussing current events, providing TV, asking his opinion on the latest issues in which he may be interested (e.g., if he has been a schoolteacher, discussing issues which concern the public schools, such as teaching methods or benefits of field trips for students, can stimulate his interest). Otherwise the patient often becomes despondent and sets very few goals for the present and future.

Pearl (12) Hearing Aid—An Improvised Alert Signaling Device

The high-pitched sound of the hearing aid can be useful. *After first removing it from the ear*, turn the volume all the way up, to alert family members or others nearby. This can suffice when the elderly person is unable to call out for help.

Before specific teaching can be effective, as the nurse caring for geriatric patients, you must create an environment conducive to teaching. A primary goal here is to stimulate and rekindle hope, trust, and interest in the often bored, despondent patient. Several means which can be used in attempting to achieve this goal are included in the following Pearls.

Pearl (13) The Family

Encourage the family's participation.

Pearl (14) What Does He Want to Do?

Assess the patient's abilities and his interests.

Pearl (15) Other Health Workers

Collaborate with other members of the health team (i.e., psychologist, occupational therapist) if available.

Pearl (16) Friends

Provide for small group projects with peers when possible (such as bingo, dominoes, hand-stitching patchwork-scraps into a pattern for quilting).

Pearl (17) A Hobby

Find a new hobby which fits his ability (i.e., the stroke patient with hemiparesis or hemiplegia may need an activity which he will be able to perform with one hand such as stamping identification data on materials or stamping envelopes, etc.).

Pearl (18) Therapeutic Diversion

Find a diversion which may also help increase the range of motion and prevent contractures (e.g., the patient with arthritis may find crumpling newspaper or tissues into balls which can be stuffed into fabric compartments to make stuffed toys or mobiles for children in pediatric units or for grandchildren therapeutic as well as diversional).

Pearl (19) Volunteers

Encourage the use of peer group volunteers (the same volunteer for the same patient when possible). These wonderful folks who volunteer can be a real help in dealing with the elderly patient.

Pearl (20) The Patient Sets the Pace

Plan nursing intervention so that the patient is not hurried and he can participate as much as possible in the decision-making process.

Pearl (21) The Clothes Make the Man

Dress the elderly person, who is on an ambulant unit, in street clothes rather than in the hospital gown. This promotes a sense of well being.

Pearl (22) Not Ambulatory Does Not Mean "Immobile"

Even if the patient cannot ambulate, when possible, get him into a chair and encourage visiting in the TV or game room for additional and often needed stimuli.

Pearl (23) Decreased Attention Span

When group activities are planned, whether they are classes in diet management, a session about hypertension, a bingo game, or a religious ceremony, it is important that the nurse remember that the elderly patient's attention span often decreases as he grows older. This is particularly important if guests are invited to lead the sessions. This should be mentioned in advance when collaborating with others in planning these sessions. Otherwise they are quite embarrassed if later in the session the older person falls asleep, wanders about, or gets up and leaves.

Pearl (24) The Lonely Meal

Almost no one enjoys having his meals alone. Conversation often stimulates the appetite. When possible, plan to visit the patients (particularly the elderly patients) who only play at eating. You will note that the food on their tray is barely touched. The volunteer (i.e., Pink Lady or Candy-Striper) or family member can be very helpful by visiting with the patient during mealtime.

THE PATIENT WITH VISUAL, HEARING OR LANGUAGE DISORDERS

Often it takes ingenuity to provide the blind, the deaf, and the aphasic patient with the nursing care measures they need. Here are a cluster of Pearls dealing with the care of patients with visual, hearing, and language deficits.

Pearl (25) Helping the Blind Person

Never walk up to and touch the blind patient suddenly. This startles him. Announce your presence by calling his name, and identify yourself. Also, let the blind person know when you are leaving his presence.

Pearl (26) No Closed Doors

Keep the room doors open. This prevents injuries caused by the patient bumping into a partially opened door, as well as by someone opening the door into the room and injuring the patient as he is nearing the door.

Pearl (27) Assisting the Blind with Ambulation

If he needs your assistance to walk someplace, let him hold onto your arm as you guide him. Never grab a blind person's arm and push or pull him across the street,

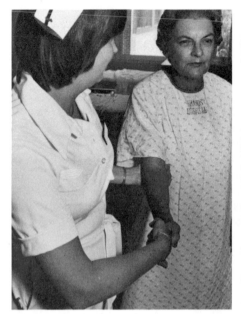

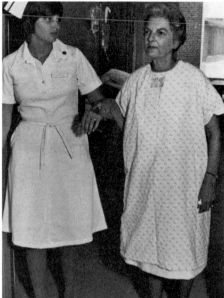

Figure 5-1   Figure 5-2

etc. First ask him if he needs assistance. (Figure 5-1 shows the incorrect way of helping and Figure 5-2 the better way.)

Pearl (28) *Blind,* not *Deaf* or *Dumb*

Remember blindness is only the absence of one special sense. Therefore, continue to speak in a normal tone and speak directly to the blind person, at the normal conversational level. Do not be condescending nor speak to him as if he were mentally retarded. It is ridiculous to try to exclude common expressions used in everyday language (e.g., "Do you see what I mean?").

Pearl (29) Ask for Patient Suggestions

When your assistance is needed, encourage the blind person to give suggestions on how you can best help in the situation.

Pearl (30) The Blindfold Approach

As part of the orientation program the nursing staff who are to be assigned to care of patients on an ophthalmology unit or patients with limited vision are blindfolded for short intervals. Being momentarily without vision while being required to perform simple tasks (such as dressing or eating) promotes a better understanding of the limitations which their patients will encounter. The staff members become attuned to real problem areas and begin planning appropriate interventions for such problems as sensory deprivation, environmental safety, diversional activities, mobility, room arrangement.

For effective communication to occur the patient with varying degrees of hearing loss must understand what others are trying to communicate. The following points can guide you in promoting more effective communication patterns in these patients.

Pearl (31) Let the Light Shine on You

Face the patient when you are speaking. Stand so the light is in your face, not with your back to a window. Note Figure 5-3 with the light behind the nurse and Figure 5-4 with the light on the nurse's face.

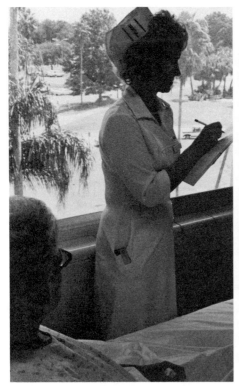 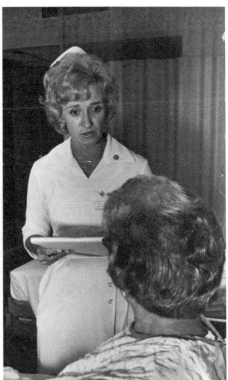

Figure 5-3   **Figure 5-4**

Pearl (32) Louder and Faster *Doesn't* Mean Easier to Hear

Speak slowly, do not shout (this distorts sound).

Pearl (33) The Deaf Person Can Still *See* You

Use hand motions, visual aids, or write the message as needed.

Pearl (34) You Rang?

The use of a hand bell is often helpful in getting the patient's attention.

Pearl (35) Too Many Speakers

It may be necessary to limit the number of folks involved in a conversation with the patient.

Pearl (36) Don't Exclude the Patient

A member of the family or other person who is quite familiar with the patient's life style and habits can be very helpful in establishing an effective communication system, initially. However, this can also be a barrier to the patient-nurse communication, if the third party is relied on too much or for too long. When this happens, you will find the third party is talking for the patient, or you are talking only to that party, thus excluding from or severely limiting the patient in the conversation.

Pearl (37) Does He *Really* Hear?

All too often, the patient smiles and nods as if he understands, but this may not be the case. Therefore, provide for feedback (by direct questioning, etc.) to assess how well the patient is hearing you.

Pearl (38) Cues for Signs of Deafness

When caring for the geriatric patient or communicating with an elderly family member, observe for signs of difficulty in hearing. Otherwise, poor communication which can lead to misunderstandings occurs.

Some cues which might make you suspicious include the patient who:

1. Frequently disregards directions (often this is merely assumed to be stubbornness without further investigation).
2. Appears to hear better when you are facing him.
3. Appears to lose interest in what others are discussing with him.
4. Tends to either mutter or speak excessively loud himself.
5. Turns one side of his head (ear) toward the speaker more than the other.
6. Often asks you to speak up.

Since decreased hearing loss is often a gradual process in the elderly, neither he nor his family may even be aware that it exists. When these cues are noted and evaluated, he should be referred for a medical examination.

Until the aphasic patient can begin speech therapy with a qualified therapist, there are several important measures which you as the nurse can employ to help the patient and his family better cope with the situation.

Pearl (39) What Is Aphasia?

Teach the patient that there are many different kinds of aphasia. For instance, this loss of language really involves one or more of the basic language skills— understanding, writing, reading and speaking.

Pearl (40) Aphasic, Not *Crazy*

Teach that aphasia is not synonymous with mental illness.

Pearl (41) Problems Concomitant with Aphasia

Often patients may have labile emotions (outburst of crying) or other personality changes.

Pearl (42) Not a Baby

Treat the patient as an adult.

Pearl (43) Give Him a Chance

Give the patient time and a chance to speak during conversations and visits. Do not interrupt the patient as he tries to speak nor become impatient and speak for him.

Pearl (44) Communicate by Caring

Do not wait until speech therapy sessions begin to start communicating with the patient. Begin establishing a trusting relationship. Be honest and thoughtful.

Pearl (45) Poor Baby

Teach the family to avoid expressing their sympathy of "how awful it must be for him" in his presence.

Pearl (46) Gear Your Conversation to the Patient

Be as consistent as possible. Use terms which may have the most significance to the patient. For instance, if he is a carpenter, use photos, objects, magazines and language that deal with his interest. Also use photos and names of family members.

Pearl (47) An "A" for Effort

Praise the patient for his efforts as well as his successes.

Pearl (48) Help the Family Help the Patient

Provide opportunities for the family to share with you or the staff their concerns, fears, and feelings. This is very important if their visits are going to be meaningful and helpful to the patient and to them.

Pearl (49) Association Rather than Stagnation

Encourage visits with others, in the day room or wherever the patient is comfortable. Isolation only promotes sensory deprivation and insufficient stimuli.

Pearl (50) Nurse, *Please!* I'd Rather Do It *Myself!*

Permit the patient to feel worthwhile. In other words, avoid doing everything for him.

Pearl (51) Speech Therapy

Collaborate with the patient's physician in order to initiate the necessary steps in arranging for speech therapy. Encourage the patient to begin speech therapy. This might require the family or friends to transport the patient to another town or care center for speech therapy.

Pearl (52) Use What He Has

Be sure to use whatever communicative abilities the patient has retained. Let him write if this is possible, or if he has a command of "yes" or "no" encourage him to use them.

Pearl (53) Bigger Is Better

Use large drawing pads rather than tiny note pads on which the patient can write.

Pearl (54) Familiarity in the Hospital

Keep familiar objects nearby; but avoid having too many objects as this can produce sensory overload and lead to confusion.

Pearl (55) Nurse, I'm *Tired*

Observe the patient for fatigue as these patients (stroke patients) often tire easily. While visiting the patient and preventing isolation are good, extended visits, too lengthy conversations and too many visitors are not good.

Pearl (56) Overstimulation from the Background

The aphasic patient tends to become agitated with background noises, or with too loud or too stimulating sounds. A visit to the day room may be helpful, but should not be prolonged. A room being shared with another patient who watches a lot of TV or listens to "blaring rock 'n roll" must be modified to meet the needs of both patients when at all possible. Bedside earphones and bedside volume controls with the volume transmitter located on each bed are helpful and often eliminate the need to move one of the patients to another room.

Pearl (57) A Picture Is Worth a Thousand Words

Often picturebooks with very few words are helpful for the patient to use.

Pearl (58) The Daily News

If the patient is used to reading the daily newspaper it may help him to be able to hold it and turn the pages, even when he cannot read it.

Pearl (59) Touching

Touching objects often helps some aphasic patient's progress. After collaboration with the therapist, continue to help the patient and his family by supporting the therapist in the speech program when the patient returns to the unit (for example, during his bath, have him touch a bar of soap then pronounce the word and see if he can say "soap," etc.).

Many aids for helping the aphasic patient can be made or bought.

VISITATION

Here are some Pearls about visits—from families, the pastor, volunteers, etc.—that help make the most out of the patient's contacts with professionals in the hospital setting. Also there are some Pearls on the important preop and pre-ICU orientation visits.

Pearl (60) A Guide for the Visitor

By providing a brief informational brochure for visitors that will make them feel welcome, and also providing a list of rules stated in a positive way (the do's rather than the don'ts), with brief explanations, many problems will be eliminated and the patient, visitors and staff will find visits therapeutic rather than disconcerting. While this information can be posted in the patient's room, it is best to make it available to the visitor at the information desk in the lobby. Some examples are 1) Check with the nurse before bringing in food to the patient. While this may be a thoughtful gesture, it may conflict with the patient's special diet. 2) Make frequent visits, but notice if the patient seems tired or restless, and then make them brief. 3) If the patient asks for assistance in getting out of bed or walking to the bathroom, when you have any question about the safety, please suggest that you and the patient first check with the nurse.

Pearl (61) The Special Visitor

The patient who is despondent due to body image alteration, loss of speech, etc. will often progress much more rapidly in his rehabilitation after a visit from someone who has made a comeback from a similar experience. For example, for the woman who has a mastectomy, or the man who is going to have a laryngectomy, the nurse will find American Cancer Society often has a Reach for Recovery or Lost Chord Group volunteer who is eager and well-prepared to make such a visit.

As the nurse you are the key person in the position to observe whether such a visit would be helpful. After collaboration with the physician, the agency is notified of this request.

Pearl (62) When Pastors Visit in the Hospital

Those ministers who have had seminary training with an emphasis in pastoral care will view their role in visiting hospitalized parishioners as one of great significance. And they should!

They have been taught to identify themselves by approaching the nursing station and generally inquiring as to the patient's status. This inquiry does not seek an in-depth diagnosis and prognosis. What is helpful is that the pastor understand the patient's general feeling and behavior over the past few days.

The pastor with clinical training has also been instructed to visit his parishioner at times other than routine hospital visiting hours. This way his pastoral work can be done relatively uninterrupted. His visit may include the sharing of the supportive rituals of faith such as prayer, or in-depth conversation such as pastoral counseling regarding the impact of the crisis of illness and its meaning to the patient.

Because this minister may have traveled more than an average distance to visit the patient or because of his busy schedule, hospital staff are encouraged to support his visit by helping to see that as few interruptions as possible occur when he is with the patient. It is most often the case that patients wish to see more of their pastor when they are hospitalized. It is the rare minister who overextends his visit or interferes with the health care professional's delivery of care.

Because the minister may have had an extended relationship with the patient, perhaps preceding the illness by several years or longer, he can often aid the hospital staff in understanding behaviors or ways of relating on the part of the patient and family. Confidential information he cannot divulge, but insights useful to the patient's care are contributions he can make to the health care team.

Hospital staff may wish, with the patient-family permission, to include the pastor in significant communications throughout the course of an illness. The pastor represents an ongoing source of help and support to the patient and family which extends beyond the walls of the hospital. As a particular minister demonstrates his trustworthiness, hospital staff can facilitate the accuracy of his work by including him in many aspects of the health care plan.

Pearl (63) Those Pertinent Preop Visits

Preop visits should be an integral part of the surgical program for the patients. Such visits when properly planned enhance communication among the patients, families, staff on the general units and the staff in the special areas (such as OR, PARR, critical care, etc.).

We believe you will find these measures helpful in implementing an effective program involving preop visits.

1. If you do not have preop visits on a regular basis, institute such a program. A staff member from the surgery units (adult and pediatrics) surgical intensive care unit (SICU), PARR, ER and the patient service representative should serve on the planning committee.
2. Identify this objective for preop visits in relation to your particular hospital situation (factors such as availability of staffing, number of surgical units, number of surgical cases usually involved, etc.). This will give you a better assessment in establishing the procedure for the visits.
3. Consider who will visit and when.
4. Plan what the purposes of the visit will be (i.e., how will the OR or PARR nurse's visit to the patient differ from the preop teaching from the staff on the unit, the physician's and anesthesiologist's visits?).
5. Plan how best to collect information that will provide the OR and PARR staff with sufficient data to give better individualized patient care.
6. Identify valuable resources such as patient and family, staff-nurse and other members of the health team, OR schedule, patient's chart and other records such as Kardex, and staff time sheets to identify which members will be available on the units.
7. Establish a tool which will be available to better transmit the information. (See the chapter on Management in the Clinical Setting.)

Pearl (64) A Visit to the SICU

Preop teaching and preparation should usually include a visit to the SICU for patients who are scheduled to return to this unit after surgery (such as after cardiac surgery). This can help decrease the high level of stress which the patient often experiences from fear of such unknowns as gadgets, a new environment, etc. The appropriate time for the visit must be planned in advance as a collaborative effort between the staff on the ward and the critical care personnel, lest the visit become a stressor in itself.

KEEPING PATIENTS INFORMED AND IN CONTROL

These next Pearls are valuable because they help us to individualize the routines of hospital life for each patient or, where that is impossible, at least make them more bearable. The secret is to provide the patient with as much knowledge and control of each situation as possible.

Pearl (65) Practice Makes Perfect

If the patient will be on extended bedrest after surgery, include in his preop teaching practice with the bedpan and/or urinal. Even a well person may have difficulty using them when lying in bed, but if the patient can learn before surgery at least he will not add inexperience to the other factors (such as effects of anesthesia, pain, drowsiness) that make it difficult to void. This could help reduce the incidence of postop urinary retention.

Pearl (66) Explain the Move

A simple but important procedure is to inform the patient that you are going to change the bed position before you touch the controls to raise or lower the bed. An unexpected change in position can be frightening and upsetting to the patient.

Pearl (67) Access to the Nurse Call Button for the Patient in Traction

For the patient on bedrest in traction, it is handy to secure the call button to his trapeze bar or to a portion of his overhead frame. This puts the call button in plain sight within easy reach of either hand.

Pearl (68) Why the Straps?

Straps of many kind are applied to patients in many different situations. These are for the safety of the patient. However, a simple explanation is often all that is necessary for the patient and his family to feel positive about the straps. When such an explanation is omitted, the patient feels and fears loss of control and being tied down. Families and patients may view this as a threatening and abusive procedure without an explanation.

Situations where straps are used include on stretchers when transporting the patient to the operating room, x-ray department, or to another unit; on the tables in the operating room, and labor and delivery rooms; and to prevent injury to the very restless, confused or combative patient from falling out of bed, or from self-inflicted wounds.

Pearl (69) A Change of Scenery

1. Change pictures on the walls.
2. Rearrange flowers or remove wilted, faded flowers.
3. Place a mirror on the wall or a bedside table that will reflect the view outside. (This is particularly helpful for the patient who is positioned away from the window.)
4. Alter light rays by changing positions of the blinds or shades.
5. Take the patient out of the same room periodically, for a walk or by wheelchair or stretcher, to the TV room or even out of doors, when possible.

These are but a few measures which will make your patient's surroundings more appealing and help to prevent boredom and sensory deprivation. These are particularly helpful to the long-term bedridden patient.

Pearl (70) Library Cart

If your hospital has the good fortune of having volunteers (Pink Ladies, Candy-Stripers, etc.) available, suggest that a library cart be organized. A cart stocked with paperbacks, magazines, games, puzzles, etc. can be brought to the patients' rooms. This provides healthy diversional activities for patients, particularly those on long-term bedrest or who simply would not bother to go to the hospital library (if one is available).

Pearl (71) Facial Expressions—Nonverbal but Communication

Remember, facial expressions, gestures, and body language send messages to the observer (nurse to patient; family to patient; patient to nurse; patient to family, etc.). Expressions indicative of disgust or pain, slumped posture, bowed head and lack of eye contact, are examples.

Pearl (72) Soothing the Hysterical Patient

The manner and approaches which are used by the nurse when intervening in the care of a hysterical patient admitted to the emergency room are very important in allaying this hysteria. Suggestions which have been helpful include:
1. Do not leave the patient alone.
2. Speak directly to the patient in a calm, firm, reassuring manner. Avoid shaking, excessive gestures, and sudden jerking movements.
3. Give simple directions. Repeat calmly, as needed.
4. Touching the patient by placing a firm (but not rough) hand on the shoulder or supporting his forearm is often reassuring and helpful.
5. If he is hyperventilating, have him breathe into a paper or small plastic bag, while you count slowly aloud to him. Instruct him to focus on trying to breathe at the rate you are counting.
6. Relief of physical pain can often be diminished even prior to an analgesic or other treatment, by the power of suggestion. Emphasize his improvement, regardless of how small. Also, the patient who is injured or sees blood or someone else injured often perceives his pain as greater than it actually may be.
7. Provide other comfort measures as permitted.

Pearl (73) Health Education in the Waiting Room

Keep health-related literature in the waiting rooms. While fiction and popular journals are entertaining, current health-related articles and brochures can serve as a valuable means of health education to the public.

Many of these brochures and booklets can be obtained free of charge from various health agencies.

Pearl (74) Patient Sit-Down Inservice

This helpful idea can be used for any patient, adult or child, on bedrest or ambulatory.

Tape to the patient's overbed table (in clear plastic folders) those things that you want to teach the patient or remind him of during his hospital stay.

Not only does this reinforce previous instruction to the patient, but it also serves as family information during visiting hours. Some topics which have been used are:
1. Why does the nurse keep asking you to cough and take deep breaths?
2. Self-breast exam
3. Leg exercises

Pearl (75) The Keepsakes

When tidying the bedside unit, do not *discard* personal items (cards, letters, photos, etc.) needlessly. When possible, store these where they will be accessible to the patient. Collaborate with the patient on which items can be sent home with his family and which ones can be discarded. The elderly patient is particularly fond of small personal items, and often loves to save everything. These personal items can help you in relating with the patient. For instance, measures such as reading to the patient, encouraging the elderly patient to reread a get-well note from a friend, displaying that favorite photo of the grandchild or of his pet where it can be seen are often very meaningful to him.

Pearl (76) Small Group Teaching

While individual patient teaching definitely is important, small group instruction also has its advantages. Assess the teaching needs of the patients on your unit and initiate small group instructions when applicable. When might you consider small group teaching?
1. When there are patients with similar needs (e.g., newly diagnosed diabetes; patients who are to be discharged on anti-coagulant therapy; preoperatively, when several patients are awaiting surgery, particularly if a similar operative procedure is scheduled).
2. When there is limited staff available for teaching all the patients on an individual basis.
3. To stimulate questions and sharing of information which may not occur on a one-to-one basis.
4. To use in conjunction with individual instruction (e.g., to demonstrate insulin injection and rotation sites to the group, followed with 1:1 return demonstration).
5. When a visual aid (film, etc.) is to be shown and followed with group discussion.

Pearl (77) The Informer

A postop problem arises, an unexpected change in the patient's condition occurs, or a diagnosis of malignancy is made. When such a situation occurs, and the family must be consulted, it is helpful to follow a few simple rules:
1. No telephoning to the family the results of tests such as malignancy.
2. Clarify the use of terms.
3. Someone should be with the family when they are told. When possible let the "someone" be a person who can follow through with the family in giving emotional support.

Pearl (78) The Family's Assessment

Provide opportunities for the family to share their reports of the patient's condition and progress. This can be done in writing as well as by verbal feedback (e.g., after visit to see their loved one in critical care and other areas; after returning from "weekend passes" or "day passes").

Pearl (79) Dispelling the Family's Fears

The treatment which the patient is receiving may have entirely different meanings for the family and for the nurse and staff. For example, a "No Visitors" sign may mean, "you are not welcome" to the family. To the nurse, it may mean, "the patient is getting that extra rest needed to recuperate." The infusion of glucose to the family may signify the last resort, while to the nurse it is a common therapy. The injection is too often viewed by the family and patient as synonymous with a *"sicker patient."*

Often by observing the family's response and offering a simple explanation, the nurse can dispell many of their unfounded fears and gain their support in the patient's therapeutic regimen.

COMMUNICATION—DIFFERENT LANGUAGES AND CULTURES

The next few Pearls deal with communicating with patients who speak different languages and have different cultural backgrounds from the nurse.

Pearl (80) Bridging the Communication Gap

Establish a list of useful terms and phrases to facilitate staff-patient communication in the clinical setting. Such lists can be prepared in advanced and later adapted to the individual situation (for instance, patients who have a tracheostomy, are on a respirator, or have any physical difficulty which limits their ability to speak). These lists can be used to make posters, charts, and/or flash cards for use by the patient and staff.

Pearl (81) Crossing the Foreign Language Barrier

Make flash cards from a list of common useful terms and phrases which can be adapted to meet the needs of the particular situation. These can be prepared in advance. The need for such language (flash) cards will vary depending on your particular patient population and locality.

One way these cards can be prepared is to invite a bilingual staff member to participate in this project. Place the foreign language term or phrase on one side of the card with its English counterpart on the opposite side (for instance, for the Spanish speaking patient: Leche—Milk).

Enclose each card in a clear plastic cover to prevent soiling. Arrange cards on a large keyring or in a shoebox. Keep it at the bedside. Disperse bright-colored category cards among the flash cards for easy reference (greetings, symptoms, food, etc.).

Another consideration which is helpful in preparing the flash cards is what phrases and terms are commonly used in that particular clinical setting (e.g., words used on an acute surgery unit which would seldom, if ever, be used on a psychiatric unit. On the surgery unit one frequently hears "the dressing," "my stitches," etc., while patient's and nurse's responses on a psychiatric unit may include "The voices tell me evil things"; "It must be frightening to you to hear the voices.").

Initially it is quite helpful to invite a family member, a member of the staff or a hospital volunteer who speaks the patient's language and English to visit the patient and the staff.

Pearl (82) Idiomatic Expressions

Just as the nurse must recognize that patients, families and nonmedical personnel need clarification of medical terms, the nurse must also become familiar with the idioms of the language of the area in which she works. These terms are influenced by cultural, educational and regional factors. For instance, to the nurse who has just moved from a small community hospital in the south to a large health care center in the east or vice versa, a part of the initial stress encountered in adapting to the new situation is often the idioms of the language more than any major differences in nursing care.

Keep a personal list of such expressions. Become familiar with their usage and meaning. This will help you in becoming more adjusted to the new location, the staff and patients.

The following table depicts a sample of these idioms which are found in our locality.

Table 5-1.   Local Lay Idioms for Medical Terms

MEDICAL TERMS	LAY IDIOMS
Delirium tremors (DT's)	Shakes
Skin irritation from heat and perspiration	Scalded, heat rash
Syphilis	The bad blood
Paresthesia or numbness of an extremity	My foot's asleep
Rhinitis	The runny nose
Convulsions	Fits
Bedridden	Layed up
Diarrhea	Bowels running off
To aid someone	To "hope" him
A furuncle or boil	A "risen"
Anxiety	Spell of the nerves
Urinate; void	Pee-pee; make water
Urinal	The duck; the cow
Anticoagulant	Blood-thinner
Barium	Chalk

AIDS IN MEETING PSYCHOSOCIAL NEEDS

Finally, as with other chapters, we end with a list of gadgets that can make the meeting of psychosocial patient needs more complete.

Once again we start with the children.

Pearl (83) Infant Bonding

The staff in the newborn nurseries, such as in the Neonatal Intensive Care Unit, are finding that the infants appear more relaxed and tend to have a greater weight gain when they can listen to a tape of maternal heart sounds and quiet classical music.

Pearl (84) A Rattle from a Disposable Syringe Casing

If you are caring for a three-month to 18-month-old patient who needs a toy, and you do not have one, here is a quick one to make from materials that are available on any hospital unit.

Take the casing from a 6 cc or 12 cc syringe. Place a colorful needle cover in the casing and tape the cap of the casing in place. You now have a rattle to occupy the infant.

Pearl (85) That Imaginative Tongue Blade

Create an imaginative tongue depressor such as the one illustrated in Figure 5-5, to aid in winning the child's cooperation for an oropharyngeal exam.

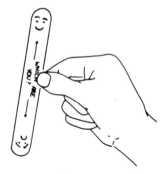

Figure 5-5

Pearl (86) Toybox

Place a toybox in waiting areas as well as in playrooms. This makes the waiting by patients and visitors with small children much more pleasant.

Be sure to include a variety of durable sturdy, nontoxic safe toys. The toys should include a variety which would be safe for children of different age groups to use. Create your own catchy reminder to post near the toybox that would help eliminate the cluttering of toys throughout the day.

Pearl (87) Plastic Mirror Toy

The use of this toy can serve many purposes. The toddler enjoys seeing himself. It can serve as a 1) diversional device for children to make funny faces, 2) for approval of self-image and 3) to help eliminate fear from dressing changes or other treatments to the face as he holds the mirror up to see himself while the treatment is being performed. It is safe, being unbreakable and without sharp edges.

Pearl (88) Funny Stickers

Use of funny stickers can be a positive reward for children. During a visit to the dentist, the children are delighted at receiving stickers such as "The World's Greatest Patient." These stickers can be used in the care of children in many situations. They can be purchased commercially or you can improvise making them on the spot to meet the needs of the particular patient's situation.

On rewarding behavior for cooperation during an injection for example, a sticker fashioned from tape and labeled in red ink, "OOUCH!" or "I AM A TOUGHIE" often suffices.

To make a supply of these to keep in stock, use adhesive tape, but back them with waxed paper to prevent them from sticking together before using.

Pearl (89) A Friendly Monitor

Infants and young children are very much in need of parental stroking. So what happens when the child's environment is frightening even to the parent? The

Pediatric Intensive Care Unit uses EKG leads with "smile" faces drawn on them to break the tension there. Parents are less threatened and more able to support their ill children.

Pearl (90) The Magic Slate

A helpful aid to provide for the patient who cannot speak is a simple slate. These slates are inexpensive and easy to use. They may be quite helpful for the patient on "voice rest" who has laryngitis and the patient who has recently had a laryngectomy, among others. It is particularly helpful to keep a supply of magic slates on the plastic surgery and ear, nose and throat (ENT) units.

Pearl (91) Quick and Simple Mobiles

Mobiles which hang above the bed are useful in helping the patient who is on bedrest cope with stress, boredom, and other such psychosocial problems which stem from long-term immobilization.

Though mobiles can be purchased in many varieties, they are easily made. They can be as simple or as elaborate in design as one desires to create. A few ways in which mobiles can be designed and used include the following:

1. *The String Mobile.* For a quick diversional toy for a child make a string mobile from various materials—colored tubing, yarn, etc. Knot varying lengths of string at several different points along a central string. In addition, the child will often enjoy making "cutouts" from construction paper or colorful pictures in magazines to attach to the strings.

2. *Personalized Mobile.* For the adult in the burn unit and other units where patients have limited mobility, mobiles which display personal memorabilia such as snapshots of family or friends or get-well cards are well received by the patient.

Pearl (92) The Color-Coded Therapy Schedule

For units, such as the rehabilitation unit, where a large number of patients are attending different therapies each day, it is helpful to place at a convenient location a corkboard which displays the entire therapy schedule. Use different colored stick pins to represent the specific therapy.

Depending on the number of patients and the variety of therapies offered, the corkboard can be modified to meet the specific unit needs. Basically, it would display at a glance *"Who* goes to *which* therapy, *when?"*

Pearl (93) Keeping Appointments

A small calendar such as a Hallmark calendar is very useful for your elderly patients and others. Assist them, if necessary, in writing in the clinic appointment prior to discharge. This is also a good suggestion for that little gift or favor when you are approached by the well-meaning friend or family member for such an idea.

Pearl (94) Syringe Container for Small Catchalls

Do not discard all of your syringe containers. Some uses which can be made of these clean containers include:

1. Tape a small syringe container to the bed, IV pole, or at the bedside. These are quite useful as individual thermometer holders.

2.   Large syringe containers (i.e., 30 to 60 cc) can be partially filled with various colored syringe container tops. Cap the large container securely and presto—a dandy child's rattle is created.

3.   Syringe containers taped at bedside can be used to keep a supply of small items, such as rubber bands, paper clips, and clamps.

Pearl (95) Pictures for Reality Orientation

When orienting an acutely psychotic patient to reality, a magazine can be useful. Have the patient identify colors, objects, etc. in the pictures. This helps distract the patient who is hallucinating and draw him back into the real world.

Pearl (96) Helping the Confused Patient Find His Way

Use wide, bright colored tape with the patient's name in black to identify his door, bed, dresser, etc. for the confused (disoriented) elderly patient. Bright colored tape helps him identify these things when he is too far away to read the name. Black and yellow make a good contrast, which is easier for persons with impaired eyesight to see. Write the name in large black letters so it can be read easily.

Pearl (97) Screening—Draping for the Modest Patient

The Screen.   What ever happened to the custom of using the simple folding screen? Curtains which can be pulled about the bed hang neatly at the bedside in the patient's rooms. But what about those examining rooms, treatment rooms, proctorooms, which have no curtains to pull and yet are unexpectedly entered by many unannounced staff members. Keep a folding screen available and use it to prevent embarrassing moments to your patients.

The Drape.   A drape should prevent prolonged and unnecessary exposure of the patient. It should prevent chilling and yet be easily manageable by the examiner during the physical examination or procedure. A bath blanket in a cold examining room helps promote psychological as well as muscular relaxation of the patient. The extent of draping will vary with the procedure and the particular individual. The nurse must become adept in assessing the patient for such needs. For example, a woman, particularly a very young teenage girl or an elderly woman, may feel more in control and relaxed if a towel is placed or provided for her to place over her breasts, in addition to being draped with a sheet.

Pearls for special problems

Unit II

Medications

Chapter six

The nurses' responsibilities in the administration of medications vary in different health agencies, but the basic principles of safety and nurse-patient interaction in the administration of medication must remain unchanged.

The administration of medication is a very meaningful experience to the patient. *How* the patient perceives this procedure as a therapeutic measure and how readily he participates in this therapy will vary, depending on the many factors involved.

The route of administration can have special significance to the patient. For instance, a visitor was overheard telling the patient, "Jim, you don't need a private-duty nurse." "Of course, I do! I'm receiving an injection twice a day," came the patient's quick retort.

Other factors influencing the success of medication administration which the nurse can often control include:

1. The nurse's approach at the bedside as she administers medication.
2. The nurse's recognition that the patient has a right to accept or refuse therapy and that this decision can often be influenced by the manner in which she intervenes.
3. The patient's ignorance of the medicine and fear of its side effects.
4. The change of dosage, time, and route of administration without appropriate explanation, etc.

The Pearls in this chapter can aid you in the safe and therapeutic administration of medications. These Pearls provide alternative approaches to the administration of medication, while adhering to the basic principles and the familiar "Five Rights" (right medication, right patient, right dosage, right time, and right route of administration).

SPECIFIC MEDICATIONS

Nitroglycerin and Nitrol Paste

Pearl (1) No Plastic for Nitroglycerin

While plastic pill boxes and bottles are easy to clean, and less likely to break, their use for keeping nitroglycerin should be *discouraged*. Why? Since nitroglycerin is a volatile agent, the plastic absorbs the active substance. Since deterioration of the drug also occurs with prolonged exposure to air and absorption by cotton, only screw-top glass containers with no cotton fillers should be used. If a filler is used that looks like cotton, the patient or nurse should inquire about this from the patient's pharmacist since some synthetic fillers which resemble cotton are used.

Pearl (2) Detecting Activity of Nitroglycerin

Teach the patient to detect if the nitroglycerin is still active. The inactive tablet will not produce the usual, a) stinging sensation when placed under the tongue, b) the relief of anginal pain, or c) headache.

Patients should discard the tablets after six months. Nurses should avoid placing nitroglycerin in a paper cup at the bedside.

Pearl (3) Accurate Dose of Nitrol Paste

Pharmaceutical companies usually supply a pad of "Dose Measuring Applicator" sheets for ease in measuring the accurate dose of Nitrol paste to be used for the patient. However, should you be without a supply of these sheets or if the patient or his family's supply of sheets is misplaced, one can be improvised by using squares of plastic wrap, wax paper, cellophane, such as bread wrappers, pieces of plastic freezer bags, etc.

Mark off inches (usually 0.5 in., 1 in., 1.5 in., 2 in., 2.5 in.) on a piece of adhesive tape in advance and stick this to the bathroom mirror, kitchen cabinet or wherever it is convenient for the patient or family member who will be preparing the dose of Nitrol paste. This will promote accurate measurement of the paste when improvised materials are used.

Pearl (4) A Psychological Hang-Up

Nitrol paste can usually be placed at different sites, such as on the leg, arm, or chest, and secured by taping the application sheet.

For reasons yet undetermined, the nurse occasionally encounters a complaint and firm insistence from the patient that the Nitrol paste must be placed on the *chest* near the heart. Apply to the chest but collaborate with his cardiologist regarding this situation for future applications. By all means try to avoid unnecessary stress to the patient.

Pearl (5) Eliminate Headache—Avoid Contact

Use caution in avoiding contact with the Nitrol paste from the previous application site and as you apply the present application; absorption of Nitrol from this contact may produce a headache.

Heparin and Coumadin
Pearl (6) Rotate Sites

The subcutaneous abdominal sites are often preferred to the arm or leg. With mobility there is less likelihood of local capillary bleeding when this site is used.

Pearl (7) Do Not Aspirate

Clear syringe of air, inject—*do not aspirate*. Aspiration causes a tendency for bleeding in the tissues at the site.

Pearl (8) No Massage

Apply pressure at the site after the injection, but *do not rub or massage the site*. This rule should be practiced following all injections. Why? Rubbing tends to produce leakage of the injectate from the site, and can produce localized bleeding in the tissues, particularly if the patient has increased capillary fragility. Any medication that needs to be dispersed on injection into the surrounding tissue should be administered with the "Z" method of administration.

Pearl (9) Special Times for Certain Meds

For the patient who is receiving Coumadin in the hospital, a daily prothrombin time is tested before it is administered. You may find that in order to have these laboratory results available, it is better to administer the Coumadin later in the day rather than with the routine daily medications which are often given at 9:00 or 10:00 A.M.

Controlled Drugs

To prevent unnecessary delay during shift changes as narcotics are counted, keep a current accurate record of the narcotics and other controlled medications administered. How? Consider the following Pearls.

Pearl (10) Sign-Out Book

Place a sign-out book in the medication room near the locked controlled-drug cabinet. Each nurse should count the amount left and see if it corresponds with the sign-out sheet for the particular medication each time a narcotic is prepared and administered to a patient.

This prevents having to search through the individual charts and/or trying to recall which patients received such controlled medications during your shift.

Pearl (11) Double-locked

Narcotics must be under double-lock and key. It is helpful to have a signal, such as a light which flashes in the nurses' station whenever the cabinet containing the controlled medications is opened.

Pearl (12) When Changing Shifts

When the nurse on the off-going shift and the nurse from the on-coming shift are counting narcotics, the nurse who is coming on duty should actually count the medications, while the nurse reporting off duty watches and both nurses check the sign-out book to see if the count is correct.

Make certain *unused* containers of these medications are *sealed* and none are missing. When there is a miscount, the supervisor should be notified and the matter corrected before the staff who are reporting off duty leave.

Pearl (13) Follow Policy

Be sure to become familiar with the nurse's role in regard to the legal aspects in dealing with narcotics and controlled drugs, as established by that particular institution and the federal control of narcotics.

Pearl (14) Pin the Key

Using a light-weight key ring, for the "narcotic" key (key to the controlled-drug cabinet). Pin the key to your scrub attire or inside your uniform pocket with a safety pin. This prevents misplacing the key.

Laxatives
Pearl (15) Perils of Laxatives

Teach the patient to avoid taking laxatives *indiscriminately*. Why? Misuse and abuse of laxatives can produce problems such as the following:
1. Dehydration
2. Chronic dependence on laxatives to relieve constipation
3. Irritation of colon and anal sphincter
4. Lack of a sensible, safe, and natural elimination regimen
5. Peritonitis; avoid taking laxatives when there is abdominal cramping (could be appendicitis and the increased motility of the intestines could produce this dreaded complication).

Pearl (16) Medications for Bulk

When medications are prescribed for bulk, such as Metamucil, *avoid giving as a dry mixture* as it can expand in the esophagus and cause dysphagia. Also, the fluid must be added at the bedside, while stirring quickly, immediately before the patient ingests it. Otherwise, it becomes a gelatinous glob and will not pour from the cup.

ADMINISTERING MEDICATIONS BY TABLETS OR CAPSULES
Pearl (17) Dividing That Scored Tablet Equally

Trying to break a scored tablet into two equal parts without success is often annoying, a waste of time and a waste of medication. Some factors contributing to the difficulty are: tablet is too hard to break by the current method used, the file for aiding the nurse in this has been misplaced, and the pieces, when broken, are not equal.

Here is an almost foolproof method for dividing the scored tablet (note Figure 6-1). Hold the tablet between the thumb and two fingers, while keeping the scoring parallel between them. Press tightly. This results in two equal parts of the tablet.

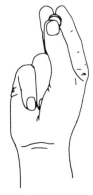

Figure 6-1

Pearl (18) Crushing the Large Pill

Some tablets are large and quite difficult to swallow. These should be crushed and mixed with water when possible. If a mortar and pestle are not available, crush the tablet which is enclosed in a souffle cup (the common paper medication cup) with a blunt object (i.e., the side of your bandage scissors).

Pearl (19) The Handy Supply of Gelatin Capsules

If the patient has difficulty swallowing large tablets, try crushing them and putting the powder into clear gelatin capsules. Some patients find that this makes medications much easier to swallow. Keep available a supply of these plain gelatin-coated capsules. When administering capsules, have the patient sip a little water before taking it. This moistens the mouth and facilitates the swallowing of the capsule. Otherwise it becomes sticky when in contact with saliva, making swallowing difficult.

Pearl (20) When Crushed Tablets *Do Not* Dissolve in Water

Large tablets may be crushed and the pieces held together with a spoon of honey or syrup.

Pearl (21) Pills and Their Hiding Places

If you suspect that the patient has not actually swallowed his pill, even though it was placed in his mouth, there are certain steps you should take to determine if your suspicions are valid.
1. Look in his mouth.
2. Examine the bed linens.
3. Check such hiding places as the pillowcase, the bedside table drawer; inside cuffs of sleeves, under the mattress, in the pajama or shirt pocket, in the flower pot or vase, etc.

The approach you should use will vary with the individual situation. You should be particularly cognizant of this problem when the patient is confused, terminally ill, or has known suicidal tendencies.

ADMINISTERING LIQUID MEDICATIONS
Pearl (22) Making a Suspension

To administer a medication which is not available in a liquid form through gastrostomy, an NG tube, or to a patient who is unable to swallow pills, open the capsule or crush the pill and place the powder in a medicine cup. Add only enough water initially to make a paste. Then add more liquid to thin the mixture to a smooth, even suspension for easy administration.

Pearl (23) Protect the Label

Pour liquid medications *away* from the label. This will prevent soiling and obscuring the label. Teach this practice to patients and family members who may be pouring a liquid medication in the home. Remember proper identification of the medication is one of the cardinal rules in medication administration.

Pearl (24) Fish-Mouthing

"Fish-mouthing" is a technique which can be safely used to administer oral medications for the patient who has no difficulty swallowing but consistently resists the necessary oral liquid medications by spitting them from his mouth. This is one of several techniques which can be used in situations where the patient should not be subjected to repeated injections (for example; the elderly patient with chronic brain syndrome who needs a laxative, sedation, vitamin supplements, etc.). Explanations regarding the use of this technique should be discussed with the physician and the family (note Figure 6-2).

Simply press on each side of the patient's cheeks using your forefinger and thumb. This holds the tongue, preventing spitting while allowing swallowing of the medication. The patient should be placed in a Fowler's position, a pillow under his shoulders, his head tilted slightly backward.

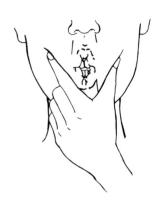

Figure 6-2

Pearl (25) Observe the Meniscus

Hold the medication cup at eye level and note the amount of liquid medication poured into the cup by reading the *lower* level of the fluid curve (the meniscus).

ADMINISTERING MEDICATIONS BY INJECTIONS
Pearl (26) The "Z" Method of Injections

This is a simple procedure which should be used more often. Clean the site, clear the syringe of air, pull tissue downward and diagonally to the site. Inject. Remove the syringe and needle. Release the tissue, allowing the injectate to be dispersed throughout (see Figure 6-3). This method is used for those substances which are irritating to the tissue. The "Z" is the manner in which the medication is dispersed *within* the tissues when the above procedure is used.

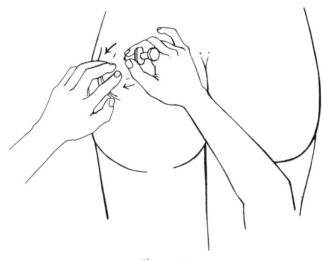

Figure 6-3

Pearl (27) Using an Ampule

Save time and endless thumping of the ampule to shift the solution from the small *upper* chamber, that is to be discarded, into the larger lower chamber (base of the ampule).

How? Hold the ampule upright between middle and index fingers and the thumb, then in an all-in-one motion, quickly raise the ampule upward and jerk it quickly downward in a half-moon clockwise motion. The downward effort should be greater than in the upward movement (Figure 6-4).

As shown in Figure 6-5, another similar method is to give an ampule a quick circular motion, while holding it upright; the fluid leaves the upper chamber and passes to the base of the ampule.

Remember, do not attempt to break an ampule without protection to prevent cutting your hand (gauze, paper towel, etc.).

If the ampule has not been scored by the company for ease in breaking at that point, keep a file on the medication cart for this purpose.

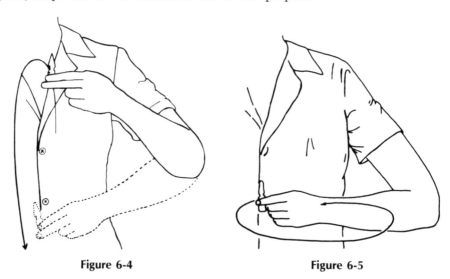

Figure 6-4   Figure 6-5

Pearl (28) Outmoded Practice

For a long time, the mixing of more than one medication in a syringe was a common practice. The medications were regarded as compatible as long as there were no obvious changes in color or consistency. Today this practice must be considered taboo unless there is absolute certainty that the medications are compatible. Critical changes could be occurring which are not detectable by the naked eye. Harmful consequences to the patient could result with the administration of such incompatible medications.

Pearl (29) Eliminate the Alcohol Sting

After cleaning the skin with the alcohol wipe prior to the injection, allow a moment for the alcohol to dry. This helps eliminate the alcohol sting at the injection site caused by the alcohol entering the site.

Pearl (30) Rotation Sites

You will find the staff is more efficient in using different injection sites if a rotation schedule is written and posted. Such a schedule should be placed for easy access to the staff, such as in the nursing Kardex or attached to the patient's medication Kardex when the unit dose system is used. In addition, it is sound practice to record in the nurses' notes the date, time, and site of the injection.

Pearl (31) Holding a Child for an Injection (10 mos to 6 yrs)

Sometimes it is necessary to give a child an IM injection even though the child is unwilling or unable to cooperate. While the technique described below should not be regarded as the common or the first approach when giving a child an injection, it is useful in certain difficult situations where time is of extreme importance. Here is a way to hold the child that involves only one nurse and the child's parent (or substitute) and *does not* prolong the child's agony with ineffective restraining techniques.

Have the parent or substitute hold the child across his or her lap, holding the child's arms firmly. This may be done with the child prone, supine, or sitting. The nurse then straddles the child's legs and clamps her knees together on the child's legs at the knee or a little above. The older child may be held easier in the sitting position. Injections may be given in the arm, thigh, or buttock.

Pearl (32) The Right Dose

To help ensure that you have the correct dose drawn up into the syringe, make a point of checking the syringe before withdrawing the needle from the vial.

Pearl (33) Checking for Burrs

Occasionally the nurse or the patient may prefer or need to use nondisposable needles and syringes. Be certain that the needle and syringe are sterilized before each use. It is also very important to examine the needle for any burrs. To check for burrs, simply pull the needle across a strip of gauze or a cotton ball. If a burr exists, it will snag.

While sterilization is important to prevent infection, checking for burrs is necessary to eliminate unnecessary discomfort or breakage of the needle during the injection.

Pearl (34) Save Medications Safely—Label

For the patient who needs only a portion of the medication from his vial, consult with the pharmacist about whether the remaining portion for the next dose can be saved safely. If so, label the vial as to the dosage left per milliliter, the time to discard if not used, and your name. This procedure should be used only when there is temporarily a limited supply available or cost of the medication is high. Otherwise it is best to discard and open a new vial each time.

Pearl (35) Rid the Air But Save the Medicine

Once you have withdrawn the medication into the syringe, point the needle perpendicular to the ceiling (straight up) when attempting to eject air from the syringe. This prevents loss of any of the medication and clears the syringe of air. Remember air is lighter than fluid and consequently will be ejected from the needle before the medication, if the syringe is held in this manner.

Pearl (36) The Right Needle

When preparing an intramuscular injection, the correct size needle must be selected. If in doubt of the amount of the individual patient's subcutaneous tissue, take an assortment of different size needles with you to the bedside. The greater the amount of subcutaneous tissue, the longer the needle should be to safely deposit the medication in the muscle. If the correct needle is selected, there should be no need to question how far to insert the needle.

SAFETY MEASURES

Be sure to consider the following measures in caring for your patients who are taking medications:

Pearl (37) Discarding Medications

Preferably on admission, and certainly prior to discharge, ask the patient and/or his family to share a list of medications which he has been taking at home. Occasionally it may be necessary to have these medications brought to the hospital.

Collaboration among the patient, family, nurse and physician must be undertaken to determine which medications must be discarded.

Encourage the patient and his family to discard leftover medications which are no longer being used. This aids in preventing self-medication of a drug which is not part of his current medical regimen. It also prevents using outdated medications that may have undergone chemical deterioration, and the sharing of medications with friends or other family members. (Remember that explanations must be given, since medication abuse is too often due to poor rationalization when the expense of purchasing a new medication is considered.)

Pearl (38) No Meds at the Bedside

Make certain that *no medications are left* with the patient unless self-administration is prescribed (i.e., as in the use of nitroglycerin).

Pearl (39) Antidotes—In Stock

When stocking the medication cart or room with medications, it is important that you include common antidotes. In event of adverse reactions, therapy should not be delayed due to the antidote needed being unavailable on the unit.

Collaborate with the pharmacist in establishing a list of the antidotes you should have stocked on your particular unit. Post a list of these to use for future restocking and for ease of locating the medication when the situation arises.

Such antidotes include: vitamin K for patients receiving Coumadin; protamine sulfate for heparin; Benadryl for allergies; narcotic antagonists; hemostatic agents such as vitamin K, etc.

Pearl (40) Lists of Compatibles and Incompatibles

Post on the medication cabinet lists of compatible and incompatible medications which you can acquire from the pharmacy or the Drug Information Center in your area. Whenever in doubt, double check.

Pearl (41) The *Right* Patient

Too often the patient may answer to another patient's name, may have wandered into another patient's room or have changed beds. So be sure to check the identification bracelet which is on the patient before administering any medication. As the nurse becomes familiar with caring for "Mr. Smith" there is a tendency to disregard this practice and the chances of error increase. The correct identification of the patient is a cardinal rule in the safe administration of medications.

Pearl (42) Emergency Drugs—On Standby

A syringe of lidocaine for "IV push" and a syringe of atropine are prepared, properly labeled and kept ready-to-go in the coronary care unit by use of wall-mounted spring-clips nearby (note Figure 6-6).

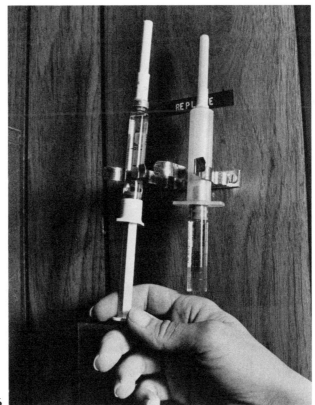

Figure 6-6

Pearl (43) When in Doubt, Check It Out

Should a patient remark that something is different about or omitted from his medication (e.g., "I've only been taking two pink tablets, do I really need three of them?" or "Nurse, is this a new tablet the doctor has ordered?"), unless you are *absolutely* sure about the change, take time to double-check with the chart, etc. Then you can reassure the patient as to the rationale of the new pills, etc.

Remember, you are usually administering several patients' medications, while the patient need only pay close attention to his own.

Pearl (44) "Sharp" Bottle

Save the disposable saline bottles to use for disposing of sharp items such as needles. These bottles are usually discarded anyway. Tape the top (as shown in Figure 6-7) for closing the bottle when it is full. These improvised bottles have been approved by our hospital's infectious control committee as safe and adequate. These save the expense of purchasing commercial sharp boxes.

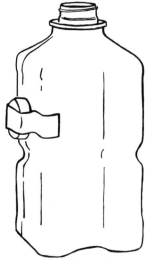

Figure 6-7

ORGANIZATION AND COMMUNICATION IN ADMINISTERING MEDICATIONS

Pearl (45) Actions of Medication—Play Role in Scheduling

Consider the action of the medication, as well as the patient's individual routine, in planning the medication schedule. For instance, when at all possible diuretics should be taken early in the day, to avoid frequent nocturia which interferes with the patient's rest at night.

Pearl (46) The Coded Medication Cart

For those medications that require withholding momentarily, until the patient is further assessed at the bedside, code them by placing a red dot or "X" in pencil in the upper corner of the card, or use another similar system. This is helpful in preventing administration of the drugs without the necessary patient assessment.

Pearl (47) File Box for Medication Tips

Keep a file box on the medication cart with specific nursing measures that are needed for certain patients requiring individualized assistance. For instance: "Mrs. Smith prefers to pour her pills in her hand rather than taking it from the cup," or "Mr. Jones (a stroke patient) must be elevated 45 degrees and turned on his right side in order to swallow his medication."

Pearl (48) Communicating the Need to Hold or Omit the Medication

Often the patient's medications will be withheld or omitted due to diagnostic tests, awaiting the report of laboratory results, or if he is NPO. Several approaches help eliminate inadvertent administration of medications. Consider the following:

1. The nurse on the previous shift (particularly the night nurse for the day shift, since this is most often the time the patient's medication is to be held) pulls and places these cards in a Hold Box.
2. The nurse (either the nurse going off duty or coming on duty) should pull these cards and clip them to her report clipboard. Therefore, as she checks her lists of duties from time to time, she will recall to check if the patients have returned to their room from the laboratory and/or if they are no longer NPO, so that she can then administer the medications.
3. If the unit dose system is being used, flag the medication Kardex with color-coded flags or a note. Be sure to remove the flag and/or note, once the patient can resume taking his medications.

Pearl (49) Unit Dose and the PRN

Keep blank three-by-five cards on the medication cart when the unit dose system of medication administration is used. By completing the medication card to accompany the medication for the patient, the essential "rights" in medication administration are continued to be practiced.

This eliminates the need to push the entire cart down to the patient's room to give him a prn medication (such as an analgesic). The nurse must avoid taking medications down the hall to the patient without correct identification accompanying the medication.

To help ensure that an accurate dosage of medication is administered by the staff, family or the patient himself, apply these following Pearls.

Pearl (50) Chart of Measurements

Post a chart of the apothocaries' and the metric systems which cite the common equivalent measures. The chart should be placed where it is readily accessible to the person who is pouring medications.

Pearl (51) Dual Calibration

Use plastic medication cups for liquid medications which display dual calibrations (i.e., dram-milliliters).

Pearl (52) Familiar Measuring Devices

When teaching the family or patient how to administer the medications, prior to discharge use common household measurements such as a tablespoon (approximately 15 ml or one-half ounce).

Pearl (53) The Tidy Med Cart

Discard trash (used med cups, syringes, etc.) into a bag (plastic, waxed or foil-lined) which you have attached to the medication cart.

A 50 cc plastic syringe *case* (attached to the cart) is a safe place in which to discard the needles. Needles should be discarded into separate containers from the other trash to prevent injury to someone who is adding trash to the bag or who is emptying the trash bag into a larger waste container.

Pearl (54) Scratch Pad on Med Cart

When you are administering medications to your team of patients take along a scratch pad to jot down requests and reminders, such as requests for analgesics (pain meds), hypnotics (sleeping pills), laxatives, etc. This will eliminate your making unnecessary trips and facilitate patient care by avoiding delays and/or repeated requests by the patient due to your forgetting the request when you return to the busy nurses' station.

Pearl (55) Medication Tray versus Cart

On large units mobile medication carts are more advantageous than trays which you must hold. They leave your hands free to assist or reposition the patient as needed. They also save searching for a clean place to set your tray, if needed at the bedside.

Pearl (56) External Meds for External Use

Store external medications separately from internal medications. These medications should be clearly labeled "For External Use Only."

Medications are seldom left at the bedside for obvious safety reasons. Occasionally a medication is kept at the bedside, such as mineral oil for the patient to apply to his dry lips. Keep the medication in a closed container (not medication or drinking cups), which is clearly labeled "External Use—For Lips." Explain this to the patient.

Pearl (57) One Organized System for Setting Up a Medication Tray

Fortunately many hospitals are converting to the unit dose system of medications. However, for some there is still the use of stock medications and, consequently, the need to pass medications to many patients from one large tray or cart. While idealistically it is safer to place each medication cup in a separate space with the individual medication card in the slot provided for that space, this is not realistic because of the lack of space on the tray when many patients the unit or on one team must be administered medications by one nurse (e.g., in functional nursing, one nurse usually administers all the medications on each shift). Various types of systems can be divised by the nurse.

The specific differences will depend on the particular needs of the situation such as staffing, type of unit, number of medications to administer and the preference of the individual nurse. Here is one example of a medication administration system which is safe and organized.

Refer to Figures 6-8 through 6-13 for clarity as you become familiar with this system for setting up a tray of medications when stock medications are used.

1. Pull the medication cards for all the patients on your team or unit to which you will be passing medications (meds) for that time period (e.g., 10:00 A.M. meds).
2. Sort the cards into stacks for each individual patient (note Figure 6-8).
3. Arrange the stacks on the tray in an orderly sequence in which they will be administered. (Usually this is according to patients' bed and/or room numbers.)

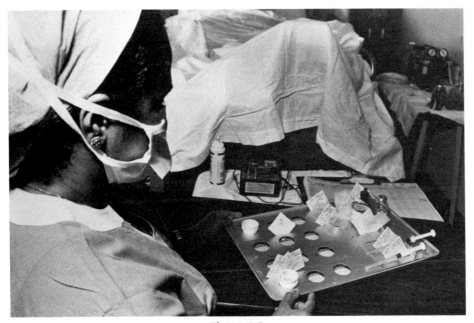

Figure 6-8

4. Begin with the cards of patient "1." For instance, let us suppose patient number 1 has three med cards for 10:00 A.M. Arrange the cards "A," "B," and "C" in the first slot on the tray so that the card at the back of the stack (C) will correspond with the last medication which is to be poured (Figure 6-9).

5. Keeping this sequence, reverse the entire stack of cards and place in the slot so that the *backside* of card C is toward the front of the tray. In other words, this stack is turned *away* from you (Figure 6-10).

6. Pull card A (which is the farthest card away from you in that stack). Place it so that the front of the card is facing forward (or toward you). It now holds an anterior position to the other two cards in that stack.

7. Pour the medication in cup A which corresponds now with card A. Place the cup so that it now becomes the bottom cup. Cup A will be the last medication to be administered to patient 1 (Figure 6-11). Each medication will go in a separate souffle med cup and the cups will be stacked.

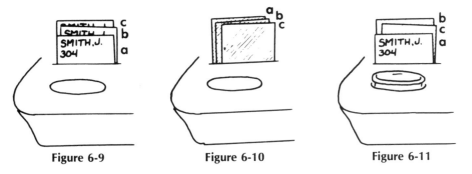

Figure 6-9   Figure 6-10   Figure 6-11

8. Repeat the same process, placing card B anteriorly to card A and placing med cup B on top of med cup A (Figure 6-12).

9. Continue the process with card C and cup C. With patient 1 who has only three oral tablets, or capsules, to take at 10:00 A.M., cup C will be the first medication you will administer (Figure 6-13).

10. As each medication is administered, reverse the medication card, placing it to the rear of the stack. This will show you *at a glance* which medications remain to be administered. It also helps you keep accurate track of which medications have been given.

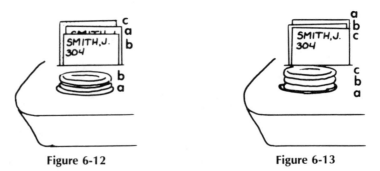

Figure 6-12   Figure 6-13

Some of the major advantages in this system are listed in the following:

1. It eliminates waste of medications due to spills from liquid medications. All liquid medications, injections, topical ointments, eye-ear-nose drops, etc. are kept in a separate section of the medication tray.

2. It saves time from searching through a tray which is not arranged in an orderly sequence to locate a particular patient's medication.

3. It is arranged so that you will more readily assess the patient regarding the need for specific meds. For instance, if patient 1 had Digoxin ordered as one of the medications, it would be in cup C and its corresponding card, card C, would be facing you at the front of the tray. This would serve to remind you to check the pulse prior to the administration of Digoxin. *Any medication that requires your further assessment of the patient at the bedside prior to its administration should be placed in such a position on the tray as described in this system.*

4. It provides an accurate check of which medications were not administered. Recall that only the cards of those meds which are administered will be reversed. This makes for more ease in charting medications accurately.

5. It saves on making additional trips down the corridor because the administration of a patient's medication has been accidently omitted.

DISCHARGED WITH MEDICATIONS
Pearl (58) Taking Meds at Home

The number of medications should be kept to a *minimum* for use at home.

Avoid complicated medication schedules for the patient at home. Correlate the medication schedule to fit the individual's routine of the day (mealtime, etc.).

Simple and clearly labeled directions for administration should be in BOLD PRINT, particularly for patients with poor vision.

The nurse should write down the instructions and clarify these with the patient and/or his family as part of the discharge plan.

Discuss examples of what procedure to follow if the patient forgets or fails to take a medication on time (overdosage can occur by "doubling up" on the medication or by taking the medication at too close intervals; also, problems can result from complete omission).

Discuss where to store the medications at home. Consider such circumstances as small children being in the home, or the patient needing to take the medication during the night.

PSYCHOSOCIAL NEEDS DURING MEDICATION ADMINISTRATION
Pearl (59) He Is a Big Boy Now
Often children will be more receptive in taking their medications if you will let them assist you in holding their own medication cups or water glasses.

Pearl (60) A Med Change
Be sure to inform the patient about any medication change (for instance, if he has been receiving a single 50 mg tablet and you must now administer two 25 mg tablets of the same medication). This is a common occurrence when the unit is temporarily out of stock of the medication and/or dosage needed. An explanation promotes trust, reassures the patient and eliminates unnecessary anxiety.

GADGETS FOR MEDICATION ADMINISTRATION
Pearl (61) Helpful Accessories
Include the following items at a convenient location on the medication cart:

tongue depressors	container for sharp needles
large drinking cups	facial tissues
carton of juice	flashlight or penlight
flexible straws	assortment of extra
	needles and syringes
Band-Aids	alcohol wipes
trash bag (water proof)	can opener

It is also helpful to take along your watch, scissors, stethoscope and a note pad.

Special therapeutic and diagnostic measures

Chapter seven

Intervening with skills and procedures is an important part of the nursing process in caring for the whole patient while in the hospital. Earlier, we discussed Pearls for meeting the *basic needs* of the patient and the assessment tools involved in physiological monitoring.

In this chapter we have included Pearls for nursing interventions that deal with the specific treatments and diagnostic measures.

It is the nurse's responsibility to see that these treatments and procedures, which become an intergral part of nursing interventions, are implemented correctly, safely and with minimal discomfort to the patient.

Tracheal care, chest bottles, and oxygen therapy are but a few of the specific therapeutic measures about which you will find Pearls in this chapter.

WATER-SEALED CHEST DRAINAGE

The following Pearls focus on the care of the patient with water-sealed chest drainage.

Pearl (1) Reliable Rule of Thumb for Water-Seal Set-up

The nurse is frequently called upon to prepare the water-sealed closed-drainage system and to change the drainage bottle when necessary.

Air is kept from backing up into the pleural cavity by placing the drainage tube under water. How much water should be placed in the water-seal bottle? Since the sizes of such bottles vary considerably, stating the amount of water in terms of quantity of milliliters is unreliable. It is best to set up water-seal in terms of the depth of the tube under the water.

Safe Rule of Thumb: Fill the bottle with enough water or saline so that the drainage tube is 1.5 to 2 inches under the water (note Figure 7-1).

As the patient breathes there is fluctuation in the water level. On inspiration the water level slightly decreases in the bottle as it rises upward in the tube. In this way, there is a sufficient amount of water for the water-seal to be maintained.

For more accurate assessment of chest drainage:

Pearl (2) Tape a Strip

Tape a wide strip of adhesive along the side of the bottle. Mark the tape at the level of drainage and initial it, also include date and time (note Figure 7-1).

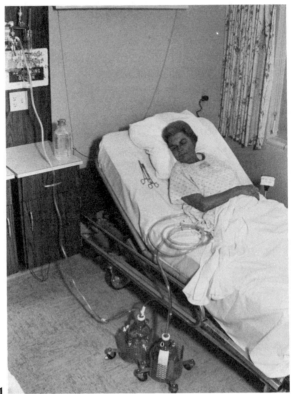

Figure 7-1

Pearl (3) No Kneeling Required

Observe the drainage at eye level. To eliminate kneeling on the floor to do this, simply place the bottle with its rack on a sturdy low stool or chair that is below the level of the bed.

Pearl (4) Accurate Record

Keep an accurate flow sheet of changes in color, consistency, and/or amount of drainage.

Pearl (5) Initial Fluid Level

If the water-seal and drainage bottle is one and the same, indicate the initial water level on the tape. This prevents miscalculations in measurement of drainage.

Pearl (6) Alert Sign

Place a sign on the room door and by the bed stressing, "Careful—Chest Bottles."

Pearl (7) Taping the Hi-Lo Controls

Patients on Hi-Lo beds must be reminded, along with the staff and others, to avoid moving the bed up and down. The danger if lowering the bed is that it can be lowered onto the chest bottle, breaking it. If raising the bed, the tension on the chest catheter can result in a break in the system (Figure 7-1).

Place a piece of tape over the buttons which lower or raise the bed, if it is electrically operated. This reminds the patient to call the staff to raise or lower the bed for him, safely. When the patient is confused or unable to follow such instructions, remove the "button-gizmo" from his reach to prevent this raising or lowering of the bed.

Pearl (8) Those Valuable Extras

Keep a bottle of sterile saline or water at the bedside should it become necessary (i.e., due to a broken chest bottle) to reestablish a temporary water-seal system quickly.

Keep a thoracotomy tray and extra sterile chest bottles on the unit.

Pearl (9) Stabilizing the Bottles, Safely

Do not tape the bottles to the floor to prevent them from tipping over. True, they will be less likely to tip over, but the chance of the bed being unlocked and inadvertently pushed aside, producing severe tension on the catheter or even pulling the catheter from the chest, is an even greater hazard.

Then how can one prevent the chest bottles from tipping over? Use special wire racks which can be obtained commercially (note Figure 7-1).

Pearl (10) Securing the Catheter and Drainage Tubing

Provide sufficient length of tubing to allow adequate patient mobilization. A trough in the sheet can be used to secure the tubing (note Figure 7-2).

The drainage tube is usually secured to the skin by sutures. For additional safety, use a 6-inch strip of 2-inch adhesive tape and apply 3 inches to the skin, wrapping the remaining free end around the tube.

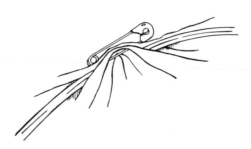

Figure 7-2

Pearl (11) Securing Chest Tube Connections

When taping the chest tube to the connecting tubing, the tape should run lengthwise and not circular around the tubing, and it should not be wide enough to completely cover the connection.

This is done to 1) hold the connection more securely; 2) make visualization of the connection possible; and 3) facilitate disconnection when necessary.

Pearl (12) Chest Tube Patency—Position Changes

The patient's position can alter the drainage and/or disrupt the system. When the patient is in a flat or semi-recumbent position, the lobe of the lung may be occluding the tube. This can be corrected by turning the patient to a lateral position or elevating to a semi-Fowler's or high Fowler's position.

Pad around the chest tube to prevent occluding when the patient is lying on his side. (A rolled towel, small sandbag, etc., can be used.) Otherwise, increased intrathoracic pressure can occur if the tubing is not patent.

Pearl (13) The Slippery Hand

Apply a water-soluable lubricant (e.g., K-Y jelly or Lubrifax) to your hands to make milking and stripping of the chest tubes easier. (When not available, lotion or powder will suffice.)

Pearl (14) Loop the Tubing

An ample length of chest tubing is necessary to provide adequate positioning and mobility of the patient without causing tension on the tubing.

However, prevent *excessive* tubing from falling to the floor as this prevents adequate drainage. Loop (without bending) the tubing and secure to the bed with a rubber band (note Figure 7-1).

Pearl (15) To Clamp or Not to Clamp

Consider this realistic but hypothetical situation: You are a nurse on a surgery unit. Mr. B. underwent a thoracotomy yesterday (your day *off duty*). You have not had a chance to read his chart. You are making rounds and notice that the visitor has tripped and broken the water-sealed drainage bottle. What would be your *first* action?

A. Clamp the chest tubes.
B. Place the chest tube in the water-pitcher below the level of the bed.
C. Help the visitor off the floor.
D. Quickly obtain another sterile chest bottle.

Considerations:
After eliminating C and D, *if* you are having difficulty in deciding between A or B, then you are encountering one of the many instances in which the nurse must make the correct decision of when to clamp and when not to clamp.

1. If you immediately select A, then perhaps you need to review the more recent information regarding this controversy. (For years, a cardinal rule was stressed: When there is a break in the system, *always clamp*, and clamp near the chest. Rationale: to prevent a pneumothorax.)

2. If you selected B, you have selected the best response *in this particular situation*. But, if you would *never clamp* the chest tube regardless of the situation, then you are not considering the rationale for not clamping in view of realistic clinical situations and the individual patient.

Rationale: *If there is increased intrathoracic pressure* (such as that which exists for a period of time after surgery, or from existing pulmonary problems), then clamping might increase this pressure leading to a *tension pneumothorax* (which can be considerably more serious than a pneumothorax). A key consideration in making your decision is what you know about the individual patient's respiratory status and circumstances. If there is known a) "bubbling" (as detected by observing the drainage water-seal bottles) or b) if the amount of suction had to be increased, then clamping should usually be avoided.

Other situations in which you may need to clamp for a few seconds: a) to check for a break in the system, b) when moving the patient on a bed from intensive care, recovery room, etc. to the patient's room on the unit. In this circumstance, if the bed does not have a special rack for holding the chest bottles below the level of mattress, and if the patient's room door is too narrow for someone to walk beside the bed carrying the bottles, then it is necessary to place the bottles upon the bed with the patient in order to get the bed through the door. (Recall that clamping becomes necessary whenever the chest bottles are raised to the level of the patient's chest or above.)

Some key pointers regarding clamping are:

1. Keep two rubber-shod clamps or specially designed chest clamps taped to the head of the bed or pinned to the patient's gown, especially if he is being transferred from one area to another. Both types of clamps are shown in Figure 7-1.

2. From the report from the previous shift, ascertain the patient's respiratory status regarding air leaks, period of time postop, amount of bubbling noted. Also read the chart and/or collaborate with the physician to find out his opinions concerning the patient's respiratory status.

3. Remember *always* and *never* should be used with caution in nursing as we provide patient care. It is better to emphasize the individual needs and demands of the situation.

Pearl (16) Shouting Over the Suction

Do you ever find yourself practically shouting as you converse with the patient who has water-sealed drainage connected to suction? Remedy: turn suction gauge from a high setting (the noise-maker) to a low setting. All that is needed is for the suction to be *on*. It is the *depth* of the suction tube below the water level in the suction regulator bottle that determines the amount of suction (note Figure 7-1).

The level of suctioning needed is usually stated in a written order.

Pearl (17) Slanted Tips

Be certain that the suction control tube and the water-seal tube has a slanted tip at the distal portion that is under water or drainage.

Smooth, rounded tips should not be used, because they become closed when shoved to the bottom of the bottle, preventing their functioning.

Pearl (18) A Checklist to Detect Signals for Action

Use the following checklist often as you assess for satisfactory functioning of the patient and his chest bottle water-sealed set-up.

1. *Check patient first.* Respiratory assessment of the patient includes examining for color changes, restlessness, crepitus due to subcutaneous emphysema from air leak; rapid, shallow respiratory pattern; or other signs of change in respiratory status.
2. *Note drainage* for a change from the last observation.
3. *Note for fluctuation* in the water-sealed bottle. (You may have to disconnect from suction to assess this.) What might be happening if there is no fluctuation?
4. *Note for bubbling.* Which bottle is expected to bubble almost constantly? Which bottle should not be bubbling?
5. *Check for patency.* What can happen if the patient is lying on his side and the drainage tube is occluded and increased intrathoracic pressure builds?
6. *Determine if a closed system exists.* What should be done if there appears to be a break in the system?

Pearl (19) The Disappearing Water Level

After carefully preparing the suction control bottle to be regulated at a certain level (i.e., 20 cm of water) as ordered, it must be checked at intervals (usually once a shift is adequate). Why? The water evaporates. Some chest set-ups depending on the particular equipment tend to have a more rapid rate of evaporation. While there are degrees of evaporation, it is gradual enough that the system is all quite safe. The following are examples of water-sealed chest drainage devices in progressive order of slower to more rapid evaporation rates if all other factors are similar:

1. *Two to three bottle set-up* (evaporation is so gradual there is seldom the need to add additional water in the course of normal use).

2. *Wall-bubbler unit, Chemetron Placement Jars* (note Figure 7-1). (May require adding water or adjusting level of tubing depth every 24 hours, and occasionally more often.)

3. *Pleura-Vac.* While it is plastic and easily attaches to the side of the bed, it usually requires additional water more often than the other devices.

When adding water to the wall suction-control cylinder (Chemetron Placement Jars), it is not necessary to unscrew the cylinder. Simply add water through the external tip of the regulator tube, or adjust level of graduated tube lower into the cylinder to the desired level.

Pearl (20) For Excess Drainage and Air

When more suction is required than the usual wall suction outlet control bottle can provide, you may find an electrical system such as the Emerson Pump very beneficial.

Pearl (21) Defoaming the Bottle

To ensure adequate visualization of the chest bottles, use a defoaming agent such as Dakin's solution (or bleach) to rinse the bottle when you prepare the set-up.

Pearl (22) Ambulating with Chest Bottles

If the patient can be ambulated, ambulate with as limited number of chest bottles in the set-up as possible. This makes mobility easier and safer.

Consider several points in ambulating the patient:
1. Where to disconnect the tubing if there is suction. Rule: must disconnect *after* the water-seal bottle. Any disruption between the patient and the water-seal

bottle will immediately destroy the water-sealed closed system. This can be hazardous.

2. Walk along with the patient with the water-seal and drainage bottle or bottles (remember they may be one and the same or separate) holding the bottles below the level of his waist.

3. If the patient is able to ambulate himself safely, place the bottle or bottles in their racks in the seat of wheelchair (which is below the waistline) and secure with tape and tie with sheet, placing towels or bath blanket between bottles to prevent breakage, if there is more than one bottle.

4. Special carriers on casters are provided by some companies (Mobile Bottle Carrier by Sklar) which will provide a mobile bottle that will not tilt. These are also used for mobile suction bottles in the operating room.

5. Rubber-shod clamps and/or an extra bottle (e.g., plastic specimen container with a cover) should also be included should a break in the system occur.

6. A mobile chest-bottle rack can be improvised by using flat wire racks (Figure 7-1) that will not tilt and taping these racks with the chest bottle onto a mobile IV pole.

Pearl (23) Aids to Removing Chest Catheter

When the chest tube is to be removed from the patient *by the physician*, it is helpful to explain to the patient how to breathe during the procedure, and to have a dressing ready.

1. How to breathe: after the patient takes a few deep breaths, the tube is pulled as he exhales.

2. Immediately, a strip of Vasoline gauze is applied over the site before the next inhalation. Tape is applied over the gauze.

3. Some physicians prefer to use only a six-inch strip of two-inch adhesive, eliminating the use of the Vasoline gauze.

TRACHEOSTOMY
Pearl (24) Tying the Trach Tube

Figure 7-3 illustrates a quick and secure way to attach twill tape ties to a tracheostomy tube. Cut two pieces of twill tape approximately 12 inches long, then cut a half-inch slit in one end of each. Put the slit end through the opening at the side of the flange. Slip the free end of the tape through the slit and pull to secure. Repeat for the other side. Then tie the tapes at the side of the neck.

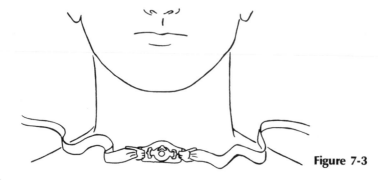

Figure 7-3

Pearl (25) Inflating the Trach Cuff

To eliminate the potential hazard of aspiration, inflate the cuffed tracheostomy balloon prior to any oral or gastric feedings. This includes administration of medications as well as foods and drinks. When at all possible, the patient should be sitting at a semi-Fowler's or Fowler's position during the feeding and remain in that position for at least 30 minutes afterwards. This helps prevent any aspiration, as well as facilitates ingestion and digestion of the food.

Pearl (26) Syringe and Stopcock

Insert a syringe connected to a three-way stopcock into the distal (external) end of the balloon cuff (note Figure 7-4). In this way a) there is better control of the amount of air used to inflate the balloon; b) there is no leakage from the cuff about the syringe; and c) there is no mistake of inflation of the balloon by inadvertent pressure on the syringe plunger as the patient changes positions or sits on the side of the bed.

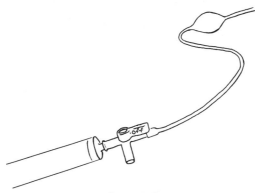

Figure 7-4

Pearl (27) Deflating Cuff

Unless a very soft, pliable balloon cuff is used (this varies with the manufacturer), the cuff should be deflated at intervals to prevent tracheal tissue ischemia and necrosis.

Pearl (28) Detecting Poor Inflation

The tracheal cuff may be insufficiently inflated if a) the patient can speak; b) there is air escaping from about the dead space (feel with palm or the back of the hand near the mouth and nose to detect this); and c) the patient is using a mechanical respirator and it is cycling erratically.

Pearl (29) Shodding the Stats

Use only rubber-shod clamps on plastic tubing or rubber tubing, or catheters. These can be used to clamp tubing such as for chest drainage, nasogastric catheters, and external ends of the balloon cuff for the tracheostomy.

How are rubber-shod clamps made? Cut two equal pieces of rubber tubing. Slide these over the tips of the clamps or hemostats so that the ridges or teeth inside the instrument tips are covered. The rubber-shod clamps protect the tubing or catheter and prevents wear and tear. Nonrubber-shod clamps can cut the tubing, particularly after being applied several times. Some companies supply special chest clamps which do not require shodding.

OROPHARYNGEAL AND ENDOTRACHEAL SUCTIONING
Pearl (30) Oropharyngeal Suctioning without Catheter Obstruction

To prevent biting of the suction catheter and promote easier insertion with less trauma to and less resistance from the clenched teeth of the patient, pass the catheter along the anterior side of the gums—entering the posterior mouth as the catheter moves across the gums at the mandibular joint area (note Figure 7-5).

This is helpful when trying to suction the confused, unconscious or resistant patient.

The advantages of this manuever include:

1. Less stimulation to the entire mouth by reaching the oropharynx using the easier anatomical route.
2. Decrease in the need to use the more sensitive nasopharyngeal route.
3. Less danger of the client biting the catheter into pieces by avoiding the passage of the catheter between the teeth.

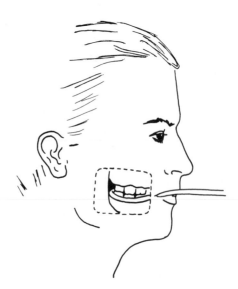

Figure 7-5

Pearl (31) Secure the Endotracheal Tube and Prevent Patient Self-Extubation

Here is a sure, secure way to tape an endotracheal tube:

1. Cut a piece of one-inch adhesive (cloth) tape long enough to go around the patient's head and overlap in the front (note Figure 7-6).
2. Cut a piece of one-inch adhesive (cloth) tape approximately eight inches long and center it on the longer piece of tape, with sticky sides together.
3. Halve the tape lengthwise approximately five inches on each end of the tape.
4. Apply benzoin to the patient's cheeks and under his nose.
5. Adjust the top half of one end of the tape under the nose and wrap the bottom half around the endotracheal tube (note Figure 7-6).
6. Reverse the process with the other end: the bottom half goes under the nose and the top half goes around the endotracheal tube several times, then laps back onto the tape under the nose (note Figure 7-6).

The tape is now secure.

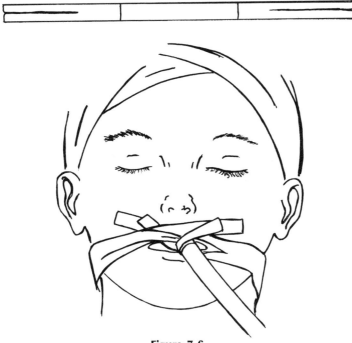

Figure 7-6

CHEST PHYSIOTHERAPY AND PULMONARY TOILET
Pearl (32) A Percussion Tennis Ball

Here is an especially good way to teach chest percussion to the parents of children who are going home: Cut a tennis ball exactly in half. It will be soft and smooth, and just the right shape to fit into the patient's palm.

Pearl (33) Chest Physiotherapy for Infants

For smaller children and infants, a nipple may be more appropriate than a tennis ball. Remove the screw-on cap from the nipple (note Figure 7-7). Pad around the rim of the nipple with cotton or gauze and "petal" it with tape or Elastoplast. Each infant can have his own in the hospital, and it can be sent home with his parents if chest PT needs to be continued.

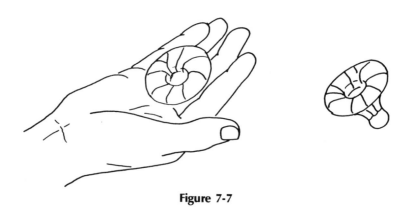

Figure 7-7

Pearl (34) Deep Breathing with a Blow Glove

For your postop patient who needs to cough and deep breathe, try making a blow-glove. You will need a disposable rubber glove, the plastic cover of a three-inch syringe and tape. Attach the glove to the syringe cover with tape as illustrated in Figure 7-8, and it is ready to blow. It is helpful to keep a supply made in advance ready to use.

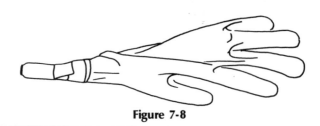

Figure 7-8

Pearl (35) Arrhythmias, Pacemakers, and Pulmonary Toilet

Cupping, clapping and postural drainage are helpful in facilitating the removal of pulmonary secretions, which in turn promotes better oxygenation in the patient. However, be sure to collaborate with the physician on this if the patient has arrhythmias or a pacemaker. It may require modifying the procedure or eliminating it altogether.

OXYGEN ADMINISTRATION
Pearl (36) How Much Oxygen? Use Safe Rule of Thumb

The exact liters of oxygen flow needed involves the determination of many variables for each individual patient. However, one general rule of thumb to guide you when you have to initiate the oxygen with no written order on the rate of flow is to apply the principle that *the farther away the oxygen source is from the lungs, the greater the flow rate that usually must be set.* For instance, a lower flow rate is usually required to main therapeutic concentrations using a catheter or mask than to operate an oxygen tent.

Collaborate with the respiratory therapy department and/or physician in your hospital for specific flow rates for various methods of oxygen administration. Keep these posted where accessible for quick reference on the nursing units.

Pearl (37) Frequent Inspection

Inspect the oxygen equipment at frequent intervals, making adjustment or repairs as necessary.

Pearl (38) Alerting Oxygen in Use

Instruct the patient and his family in the essentials of oxygen use. An important factor in successful oxygen therapy is the cooperation of the patient. Post signs at the bedside and on the patient's door, warning "No Smoking—Oxygen in Use."

Be sure to inform other patients who may be in the room and visitors that oxygen has been started and is presently in use.

Pearl (39) How Much Oxygen?

Because the liter flow is not an accurate guide to the actual percentage of oxygen in the inspired air, a chemical analysis should be done periodically. Such equipment is provided with detailed instructions for operation. The process of making the analysis is a simple one but very important to ensure adequate oxygen therapy.

If a cylinder of oxygen is used, a special gauge on the regulator should be used to indicate the amount of oxygen supply left in it.

Pearl (40) Discontinue, Gradually

When patients have had oxygen therapy over an extended period of time, it must be discontinued *gradually.* Usually the higher the concentration of oxygen, the more gradual the reduction and termination should be.

The following Pearls concern the care of the patient in a tent.

Pearl (41) No Oil or Alcohol

Avoid a potential fire hazard by using a lotion instead of oil or alcohol for the patient's back rub.

Pearl (42) Electrical Devices

Substitute other devices for electrical ones, such as a hand bell instead of the electric call light or a hot water bottle rather than a heating pad.

Pearl (43) Sealing the Canopy

Keep the canopy tucked well under the mattress. Seal the free edge with a bath blanket or draw sheet.

Pearl (44) Cover Shoulders

To prevent chilling, particularly for the febrile patient, cover the patient's shoulders with an extra wrap (e.g., a towel).

Pearl (45) Bubbling Is Patency

Check the patency of the oxygen prongs or catheter, as they can become occluded from dried mucus. Check for patency by placing the catheter tip or prong tips in a cup of water and observe for the occurrence of bubbling. This indicates the catheter and/or prongs are patent (note Figure 7-9).

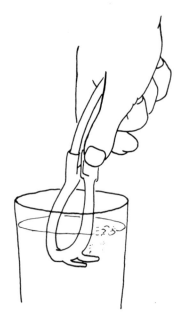

Figure 7-9

Pearl (46) The Oxygen Catheter

Use only a water-soluble lubricant when inserting an oxygen catheter. Determine the natural droop of the catheter (see Figure 7-10; Figure 7-11 shows the incorrect manner of holding the catheter). Elevate the tip of the nose and pass the catheter through the nasal orifice, *with* the oxygen flowing, using the position of the catheter's natural droop. Pass the catheter along the floor of the nose. This corresponds with the individual's anatomical nasal structure and prevents unnecessary trauma to the tissue.

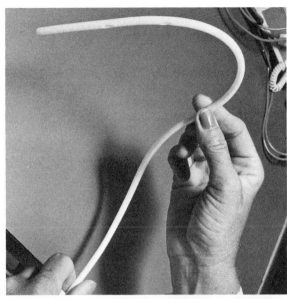

Figure 7-10 (top)
Figure 7-11 (bottom)

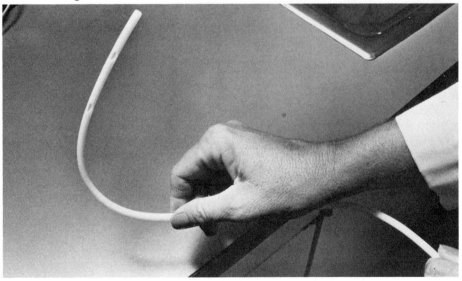

Pearl (47) Humidification—Is It Necessary?

It is important to provide a sufficient amount of moisture in inspired air. Often when initiating the oxygen therapy, the nurse is confronted with the decision of whether to provide a source of humidity (such as a container of water at the oxygen outlet through which the gas can pass).

Some points to guide the nurse in the decision include:

1.   If the oxygen passes through the nose (as with nasal prongs, face masks,

etc.), saturation level with natural humidificaton is sufficient by the time it reaches the trachea.

2. If the oxygen by-passes this natural humidification of the nose (as with nasal catheter which extends to uvula, tracheostomy adaptor, etc.), a container of water connected at the oxygen outlet (or by other means of mechanical humidification) must be provided through which the oxygen can pass.

TREATMENT AND ASSESSMENT OF THE GENITOURINARY TRACT

The following Pearls deal with those diagnostic and therapeutic measures used in the assessment or treatments associated with the patient's genitourinary system.

Pearl (48) Catch the Urine in a Bowl

Here is how to make measuring output easy for the ambulatory female patient (and the nurse who cares for her). Place the collecting bowl in the inner part of a hanger which has been bent to fit it, and suspend the bowl in the commode beneath the front part of the toilet seat (note Figure 7-12). Now the patient can use the commode freely, and yet save her urine.

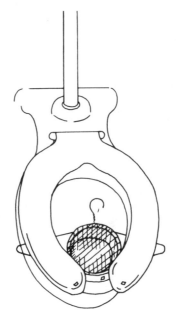

Figure 7-12

Pearl (49) The Straight Streamer

The straight streamer is a plastic device which can be used by the woman as an aid in collecting clean-catch urine specimens (Figure 7-13). This device is particularly useful in clinics. A chart of step-by-step instructions on how to use the streamer is placed in the bathroom. This mid-stream catch device was developed by Robert Cade, M.D.

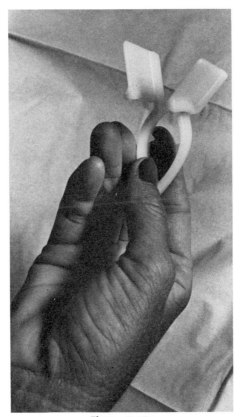

Figure 7-13

Pearl (50) Instructions for Straight Streamer

Clean catch (A chart with following illustrations and instructions are posted by the toilet.):

1. Undress from waist down.
2. Stand facing the toilet with legs spread apart.
3. Carefully unscrew the cover of the urine container, being certain to avoid touching the inside of either lid or container. Now place lid (inside up) and container on the shelf beside you.
4. With the index and middle finger, spread the lips (labia) that cover the urinary opening (meatus) wide apart.
5. Note how to hold the device (Figure 7-14). Continue holding the lips (labia) apart and with the other hand grasp the device and squeeze the wings of the urinary device together.

6. Still squeezing the wings together, push the pointed end of the urine device fully into the vagina (Figure 7-14).
7. Remove the hand, holding the lips (labia) apart. Slowly release the wings of the device. The device should now be open and holding the lips apart (Figure 7-15).
8. Remain standing and begin to urinate into the toilet.
9. Bring the urine container into the urinary stream catching the urine in the container. Place the container down on the shelf and finish urinating into the toilet.
10. Carefully replace the cover on the container.
11. Squeeze wings of urine device again together and carefully remove it.
12. Pat dry with tissue and replace your clothing. Give the device and container of urine to the nurse.
13. *If you cannot* urinate standing, then be seated on the toilet with legs spread widely apart and proceed with the instructions beginning with number 4.

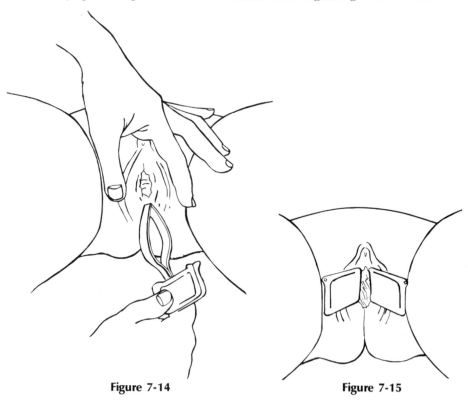

Figure 7-14   Figure 7-15

Pearl (51) A Problem with the Urinary Catheterization of Females

When there is difficulty locating the meatus: use additional lighting (e.g., portable goose-neck lamp) and lift the patient so that her hips are on an upside down bedpan or put the patient on an exam table with feet in stirrups. Then *gently* probe each dimple with a sterile Q-tip until the meatus is located.

Pearl (52) Leave the Catheter to Prevent a Second Error

When inserting a urethral catheter in a female patient, if on first attempt the catheter ends up in the patient's vagina, leave the catheter there rather than removing it before you try again. This will provide you with an additional landmark so that you do not repeat the error.

Pearl (53) Getting That Scarce Drop of Urine for a Specific Gravity or Other Test

This Pearl is a useful way of getting a few drops of urine from a premature or otherwise very small infant, who is *not voiding enough to soak a diaper*. (A diaper must be quite wet in order to wring out a drop of urine needed for a specific gravity or dipstick.) Note: This method is only useful with a *disposable* diaper (see Figure 7-16).

1. Remove a small piece of the absorbent inner liner of the diaper, which is the most saturated area.
2. Place this lining within the lumen of a 3 cc or 6 cc syringe.
3. Replace the plunger and inject the drops of urine where they are needed to perform the test.

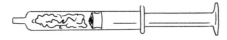

Figure 7-16

Pearl (54) Culturing the Catheter Tip

For a better chance of having a more reliable specimen, try these suggestions the next time the indwelling urinary catheter tip is to be sent to the laboratory for a culture.

1. Gather these supplies which are needed for removing the indwelling catheter:
   a. A Chux or other pad to prevent soiling the linen.
   b. Sterile gloves and a gauze sponge; or sterile applicators.
   c. Culture tube with a large enough diameter for placement of the catheter tip.
   d. Sterile scissors and thumb forceps (usually part of the dressing or suture kit).
   e. Antiseptic agent.
   f. A clean container sturdy enough to hold the culture tube during placement of the catheter tip into the tube.
   g. Correct size sterile syringe for removing solution in the balloon.
2. Collect any urine specimen needed before removing the catheter.
3. Deflate the balloon to the indwelling catheter with the syringe.
4. Cleanse around the meatus and the catheter with the antiseptic agent (using gloves and sponge or the saturated applicators) being careful to avoid removing the catheter until you are ready to do so.
5. Remove the catheter without contaminating the tip.
6. Using the sterile forceps, grasp the catheter approximately two inches from the tip, placing approximately one inch of the tip within the culture tube. Using the sterile scissors, cut catheter tip so that it falls within the culture tube.
7. Place the cover on the culture tube, label and send it promptly to the laboratory.

Pearl (55) Streamline Diabetic Urine Testing

When instructing the patient to test his urine for sugar and acetone, while he is still in the hospital, be sure his equipment is all located in one place by the sink, and tape a color chart at the sink where he will be testing his urine. Provide him with a chart and advise him to continue this practice after discharge. This will help improve both patient compliance and accuracy.

Pearl (56) An Essential Match

For accurate results on testing the patient's urine for sugar and acetone, the specific posted color chart and the directions for testing must correspond with the specific tablets or tape used. Therefore, when a different method is used double check to ascertain that the proper supplies are available.

Pearl (57) The Protected Slide

Points to practice for better specimens when using a prepared slide to send to the laboratory for diagnostic study include:
1. Place a paper clip on the edge of the slides to prevent the slides from sticking or other movements which can disrupt the specimen.
2. When available, use the special specimen containers for slides which have grooves to prevent untoward movements of the slide or slides.
3. Cover the entire slide with the fixation agent (a formalin-alcohol mixture, etc.).
4. Spray slides with inexpensive hair spray. This protects the specimen without having to bother with liquid fixative agents.

Pearl (58) A Speculum Warmer

A relatively new idea that is catching on in many women's clinics is using a heating pad set on low as a speculum warmer. We have received much positive feedback about this from women who have had previous exams with an icy cold speculum!
1. If speculums are kept in a drawer, use the heating pad as a liner in the bottom of the drawer.
2. If speculums are out on a table, lay them on half of the heating pad, and cover them with the other half. The speculum may become too warm as the day goes on, so it may be necessary to line the heating pad (with a pillowcase for example).

Pearl (59) Use of T-S Meter

The T-S meter can be used to measure specific gravity from scant amounts of urine (minimum 2 drops) and to determine serum solids.

Two drops of urine are placed on the meter slide (note Figure 7-17). The plate is dropped down onto the urine and slide. The meter should be held up to a light source and the specific gravity is read on the left-hand scale.

To determine serum solids, you need a sample of the patient's plasma. An easy source is to spin a hematocrit (HTC) and break the capillary tube and drop a small amount of plasma on the meter slide. Drop the plate down on the plasma. Hold the meter up to a light source and read the serum solid on the right-hand scale.

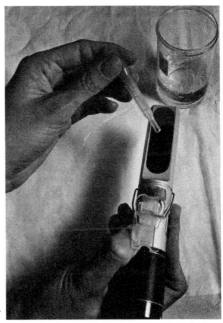

Figure 7-17

HYPOTHERMIA
Pearl (60) Sponging
When sponging is necessary to aid in reducing fever, place cold wet compresses near arterial sites (groin, side of neck, popliteal fossa, behind the knees, and also under the arms). Change the compresses frequently. Also rub the compresses briskly but lightly over the body. These measures aid in more quickly reducing the temperature.

Pearl (61) The Cooling Blanket
When the hypothermia machine with cooling blanket is used, be sure to check the patient's temperature often (using a regular thermometer periodically as well as the automatic rectal temperature probe). Avoid' setting the desired temperature control too low. Remember, too rapid reduction of temperature can produce dangerous complications such as arrhythmias. Also the temperature usually will drift as much as a degree lower than set on the machine.

Pearl (62) Refrigerate the Glove
Keep gloves three-quarters full of water, frozen in the refrigerator. It saves time in preparation where they are needed. These gloves are helpful for many uses, such as in decreasing edema at the former infusion site, decreasing scrotal edema, and preventing edema after procedures such as arteriograms. (Remember to protect skin from ice burn by placing a small wrap such as a washcloth or towel about the frozen glove.)

Pearl (63) A Five-Fingered Ice Pack

Here is a quick, one-time use, disposable ice pack: Fill a disposable latex glove with small cubes or crushed ice, tie the opening, and wrap it in a washcloth. This involves minimal expense, minimal time spent, and all the supplies are available to you on your unit. Also, the ice pack made in this way is not as heavy as most commercially available products.

Pearl (64) Easy Method to Fill the Ice Bag or Ice Collar

When an ice bag or ice collar needs to be filled with ice, make the task easier by placing a paper cup (which has the bottom removed) into the top or neck opening, of the collar and then add the ice through the cup. This permits faster filling (note Figure 7-18).

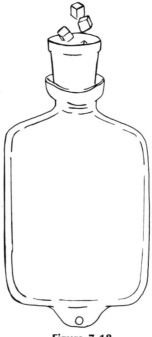

Figure 7-18

DRESSINGS

Dressings, binders, and securing tubing are approached in the Pearls which follow.

Pearl (65) For the Occlusive Dressing

When an occlusive dressing is needed such as for fresh postoperative incisions or subclavian lines for hyperalimentation, it is important that the dressing be applied securely with minimal irritation to the skin in the surrounding area. The method of application should include:

1. Using a sterile applicator, apply a small margin of tincture of benzoin to the skin about the edges of the dressing (note Figure 7-19).

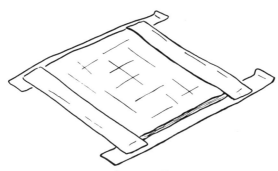

Figure 7-19

2. After allowing to dry briefly, until the skin is tacky to touch from the benzoin, encircle the edges of the dressing with tape so that one-half of the width of the tape overlaps onto the tacky skin (note Figure 7-19).
3. Then cover the dressing completely with the strips of tape by placing the strips across dressing, overlapping only the tape that encircles the dressing (note Figure 7-20). This eliminates excessive taping of the skin and yet provides a secure occlusive dressing.
4. Use of sterile technique throughout each step of the procedure.

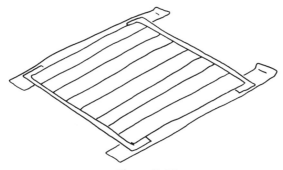

Figure 7-20

Pearl (66) A T-Binder for Perineal Dressings

Following perineal surgery such as a perineal prostatectomy or an abdominoperineal resection, dressings are held in place by a T-binder. When the patient is to be out of bed at intervals, this binder will fit more securely if it is applied while he is standing (note Figure 7-21). This helps eliminate additional adjustments later.

The dressing should be applied so that it a) does not produce tension on an indwelling Foley catheter, and b) supports the scrotum. The preferred, disposable T-binders are now available commercially (note Figure 7-22).

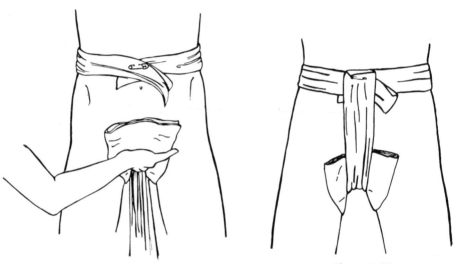

Figure 7-21   Figure 7-22

Pearl (67) How to Apply the Perineal Dressing

For patients with moderate to profuse drainage, use a *heavy dressing pack*, which includes a heavy dressing (ABD pad), as the outer layer. Then add several four-by-four gauze squares as and inner layer.

1. When possible, have the patient stand (with feet comfortably apart).
2. Place T-binder about his waist and secure it with a safety pin.
3. Place the perineal dressing.
4. Secure the dressing by bringing the posterior tails of the binder to the waistline. When preferred, the binder may also be applied lower across the abdomen rather than at the waistline.

Pearl (68) Montgomery Straps

For those abdominal dressings which need to be changed often, secure the dressing by using strips of tape known as Montgomery Straps. (These can also be purchased commercially.)

Pearl (69) To Make Montgomery Straps

1. Cut six-inch strips of two-inch tape. The size of tape will vary depending on the size of the patient and the type and amount of bulky dressing.
2. Make a two-inch fold at one end of the strip.
3. Cut a small slit in the center of the folded end of tape.
4. Gauze or umbilical tape can be used as ties to be threaded through the slits (see Figure 7-23).

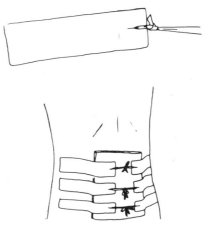

Figure 7-23

Pearl (70) Application of Montgomery Straps

These Montgomery Straps should be applied so that strips overlap each other as they crisscross the abdomen. Therefore, only one to two safety pins are needed to secure the binder. Begin at the lower edge of the binder and progress upward.

Pearl (71) The Many-Tailed Binder

Applying the dressing over the abdominal surgical incision in a patient who has a pendulous abdomen will aid in preventing infection. However, dehiscence and evisceration can occur if the abdominal muscles have poor tone and there is resulting tension on the sutures.

If correctly applied, a scultetus (many-tailed) binder can be used to prevent tension on the suture and help decrease the discomfort in these patients.

The binder has several tails (usually five) each of which, as it attaches to the body of the binder, overlaps one-half of the one (strip of fabric or tail) below it.

How to apply the binder:

1. Place the body (center of the binder) lengthwise under the patient. It should be placed so the lowest tail crosses over the extreme lower abdomen (note Figure 7-24).
2. Its placement should not interfere with any perineal drainage, bowel movement or the patient's voiding.
3. The tails are brought one by one from either side, crossing obliquely over the abdomen at the midline.

4. The binder is applied to give firm support. How comfortable it is to the patient will determine how snugly it should be applied.
5. The binder is usually applied from below upward, with the lowest tails being applied first.
6. Check to eliminate wrinkles and keep the tails from causing pressure over bony prominences.
7. When the last tail is wrapped over the abdomen, secure the binder ends with safety pins at the waist (note Figure 7-25).

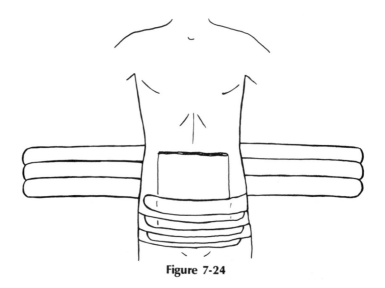

Figure 7-24

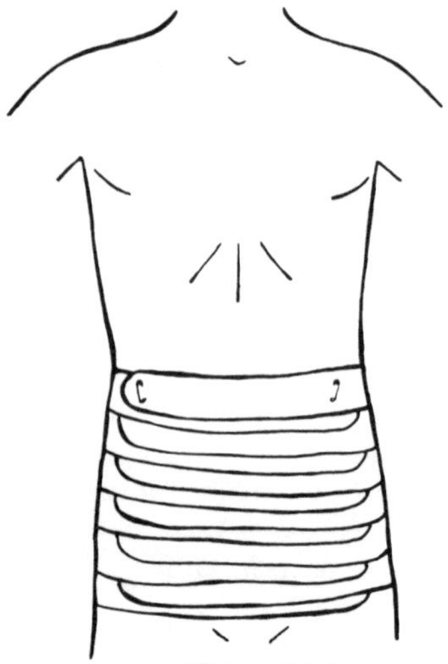

Figure 7-25

SECURING AND RETAINING TUBING, ENEMAS, AND FISTULAE
Pearl (72) Taping the NG Tube

A *correct* way to secure the nasogastric tube to prevent it from slipping is depicted in Figure 7-26. Two other techniques are commonly used for securing the tube. These have definite drawbacks which the correct technique avoids.

In the one incorrect technique (Figure 7-27), there is tension from the pull on the tube against the lateral wall of the nostril. This causes excoriation and can be quite painful in just a short time.

In Figure 7-28, there is often tension to the superior wall of the nostril. Also, if you place your finger so that it rests on your forehead between your brows, you can readily see that in addition to the tension it makes the patient feel as though his eyes are becoming crossed.

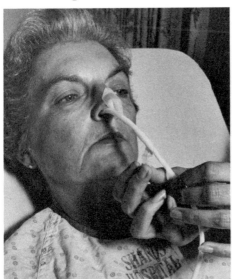
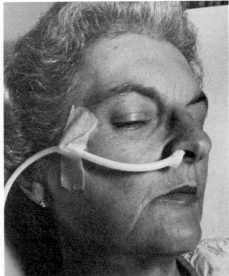
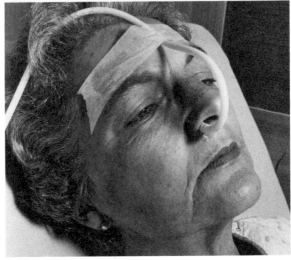

Figure 7-26 (top left)
Figure 7-27 (top right)
Figure 7-28 (bottom)

Pearl (73) How to Apply the Tape Correctly

Refer to Figure 7-26 for the correct method of applying the tape.
1. Clean the skin on the nose by using adhesive remover.
2. Cut a three- to four-inch piece of tape which is one to one and a half inches wide. (This varies with the width of the patient's nose.)
3. Cut the tape, dividing it lengthwise, leaving a one-inch margin undivided at one end.
4. Place the end with the one-inch margin securely across the nose.
5. Take the divided ends of the tape and wrap one clockwise around the tubing and one counterclockwise.

Your patient will find this much more comfortable than the methods illustrated in Figures 7-27 and 7-28.

Pearl (74) Cannulating High Pressure Arteriovenous Fistulae

Situation: high-pressure AV fistulae (large bore bovine, Gortex, or even autografts) have been known to push the plungers out of syringe barrels, or even push needles out of the AVF itself.

Solution: Always place a hemostat on the cannulation needle tubing *prior* to insertion. When the needle is in place, tape it as depicted in Figure 7-29. This will hold the needle steady and prevent it from being pushed out of even the highest pressure AVF's.

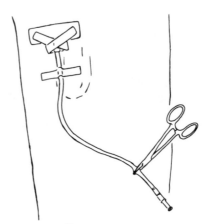

Figure 7-29

Pearl (75) Retaining the Enema

Three measures which have proved effective aids in the retention of the enema, allowing the patient to receive its desired therapeutic effect, are:
1. Apply a rolled wash cloth against the anus with slight pressure.
2. Raise the foot of the bed.
3. Encourage the patient to take slow deep breaths and gently massage the abdomen as the enema is being instilled.

STIMULATING THE ROOTING REFLEX
Pearl (76) The Rooting Reflex

As the new mother begins to breast feed her newborn, there can be anxious moments when trying to get the baby to nurse. If the baby does not nurse right away, teach the mother to first place the infant's cheek against her nipple. This should initiate the infant's rooting reflex and the infant can begin nursing.

OPHTHALMIC TREATMENTS
Pearl (77) Everting the Eyelid

Occasionally it is necessary to evert the eyelid (e.g., to apply medication directly to the inner side of the lid, also to remove a foreign object from the inner lid). Figure 7-30 illustrates how to evert the lid.

With clean hands, grasp the lashes and exert pressure on the center of the upper lid with a cotton applicator. With a gentle pull upward on the lashes, the lid will evert up over the applicator.

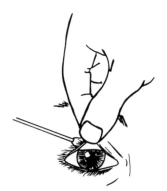

Figure 7-30

Pearl (78) Tilt Head

Have the patient tilt his head slightly back and to the side as you place the drops gently into the conjunctival sac—never with force on the eye itself.

Pearl (79) Occlude the Duct

To prevent medication from draining into the lacrimal duct, have the patient hold a sterile gauze sponge at the inner canthus. This is to prevent loss of some of this medication through the duct which would result in less than the desired dose needed.

Also, with some ophthalmic agents which are allowed to flow toward the inner canthus and through the lacrimal duct, there is a potential for a rapid systemic response resulting in possible untoward side effects.

Pearl (80) A Lateral Approach

To help prevent the patient from blinking as you start to administer the eye drops, approach the eye from the side or from below rather than from above or directly in front of the eye.

Pearl (81) Clipping Lashes

As you clip lashes, to prevent the loose lashes from falling into the eye, have the patient close his eyes and clip the lashes with scissors which are lubricated with sterile lubricant (e.g., Lubrifax, or K-Y jelly).

Clipping of lashes is usually done (preoperatively) to decrease the possibility of introducing infection into the eye.

Pearl (82) After Eye Surgery

To prevent increased intraocular pressure after eye surgery, certain basic rules are a must:

1. Prevent constipation, as straining can increase the intraocular pressure.
2. Teach the patient to avoid rubbing his eyes. Initially the eye should be covered at all times. A protective shield is used day and night shortly after surgery. Later, glasses can be worn in the daytime, but the shield should be worn at night. (Petal the edges of the shield for comfort and prevention of irritation to the skin.)
3. Avoid heavy lifting. It is best if someone can assist with the care of any small children who are in the household until after the return check-up, in order to prevent having to stoop and lift the child and to avoid sudden movements. Pets should also not be underfoot during this early recovery period.

Prevent undue concern by mentioning to the patient the common visual limitations he may expect to experience at first.

Pearls used in removing corneal contact lens from a patient, who is either unconscious or conscious, follow.

Pearl (83) Use Penlight

First locate the lens by using a small flashlight or penlight; shine it in the eye from a side angle.

Pearl (84) Check for Medi-Alert

If an unconscious patient is admitted through the emergency room, ask the family if he wears contact lenses or check for such a medi-alert identification card as you assess his condition.

Pearl (85) Handy Suction-Cup

Keep a small suction cup contact lens remover for ease in removing contact lenses in the clinic or emergency room.

Pearl (86) How to Remove Lens

To remove a corneal contact lens from an unconscious patient, see Figure 7-31 and the following instructions.

1. Place one thumb near the edge of the upper lid and the other thumb near the edge of the lower lid.
2. Place the lens over the cornea corner, if it has been displaced, sliding it with a gentle movement of the thumb on the lids.
3. Widen the eyelids above the top and below the bottom of the lens.
4. Press the eyelids *gently* on the eye until the eyelids touch the lens edges.
5. Press with slightly more pressure on the bottom lid, sliding it under the lens.
6. Move the eyelids toward each other, gently sliding the lens out.

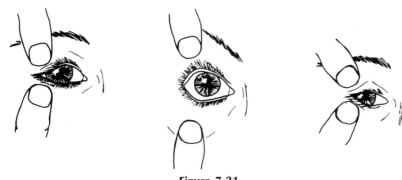

Figure 7-31

Pearl (87) When Contacts Are Difficult to Remove

Never try to remove contact lens with cotton applicators, tissues or fingernails. If you cannot remove the lens, slide it onto the sclera and call for someone more experienced with this.

If the patient is in the emergency room or is being transported to another area, and you did not remove the lens for whatever reasons, place a piece of adhesive on the patient's forehead labeled, "Check contact lenses."

Pearl (88) No Pressure on the Eye

Whether there is hemorrhage from the eye, or if one is simply opening the lids wider to place drops or cleanse the eye, *no pressure should be placed on the eye itself.* This can lead to increased intraocular pressure and do irreparable damage.

Also avoid rubbing the eye. (For example, when the child gets soap in the eye, do not rub with a cloth but rinse with lots of water.)

Pearl (89) Preventing Corneal Ulceration

For those patients with neurological disturbance in which one or both eyes remain open, tape a small Telfa square over the eye, using paper tape. Lubricating drops in the eyes are also helpful. Consult with the physician about the choice of drops.

Pearl (90) Polliwogs

Eye sponges are tapered at each end for collecting blood and other drainage from the operative field during ophthalmic surgery. These "polliwogs" can be made in advance and kept sterile.

Pearl (91) How to Make Polliwogs

1. Wash the powder from your gloves by rinsing them thoroughly in a sterile splash basin.
2. Place small sterile cotton balls in a container of sterile water.
3. Then roll the sponges one at a time between your gloved hands.

Physiological monitoring

"How's the patient?" "Nurse, how am I doing?" are questions frequently asked of the nurse. They express the real concern about the patient's condition of the staff, the family, and the patient himself. This chapter focuses on the Pearls that deal with those crucial observations of physiological monitoring, known as the *Vital Signs:* temperature, pulse, respiration, blood pressure and other interrelated observational data.

USE OF THE EQUIPMENT IN PHYSIOLOGICAL MONITORING
Pearl (1) A Change in the Procedure

The nurse must recognize there is a distinct difference between *altering a procedure* to meet the individual demands of the immediate situation, and *changing the procedure haphazardly and carelessly.*

Far too often the more frequently used procedures are abused. When improvisations must be made, they should be made based on sound rationale. This is important for obtaining the desired and most reliable results.

If one becomes slipshod in the application of standard procedures, after a period of time it may be difficult to recall the correct procedure.

An example of a commonly abused procedure is the use of the cuff and sphygmomanometer to obtain blood pressure. Obtaining incorrect information with this procedure is often due to the failure of the staff to consider such steps and rationale of the procedure as the following:

1. Is the correct cuff size being used?
2. Is it correctly applied?
3. Did you palpate the pulse prior to inflating the manometer?
4. Are you producing unnecessary discomfort from overinflating the cuff? One should continue to inflate the cuff only 30 mm/Hg pressure above the manometer reading at the point the pulse was obliterated.

5. Are you having to reinflate the cuff due to a) faulty equipment; b) deflating the cuff too rapidly (deflate at rate of 3 mm/Hg/sec); c) failure to place the manometer so that it can be visualized for a clear, accurate reading?

Pearl (2) Cold Stethoscopes Can Be Shocking

A very thoughtful thing to do for a patient is to warm the stethoscope in the palm of your hand before placing it on his chest. A change in pulse and respiratory rate could result for a few seconds from placement of a cold stethoscope on a patient.

Pearl (3) The Right Size Cuff for the Obese Patient

It is important to have several sizes of blood pressure cuffs on hand. Accurate blood pressure readings cannot be obtained when an incorrect size cuff is used. For example, if the cuff used for the average size adult is used on the very obese patient, you will obtain an inaccurate reading which is usually elevated. One could misinterpret the findings as indicative of hypertension.

Some manufacturers now sell their sphygmomanometer along with three different sizes of cuffs.

Pearl (4) Reversing the Blood Pressure in the PARR

In many instances, the nurse in the recovery room finds it is necessary to provide much of the care to the patient, which requires using much equipment and positioning near the head of his bed (having to suction frequently, check pupils, provide oxygen, etc.). In such situations, the nurse will find it easier to invert the blood pressure cuff so that the readings can be taken while it is necessary to care for the patient from this angle (note Figure 8-1).

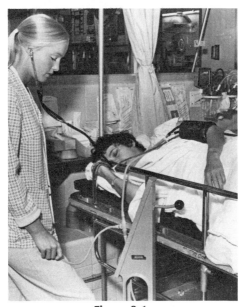

Figure 8-1

Pearl (5) Stethoscope for Anesthesia Cuff

Observe Figure 8-2 for how the staff in our PARR make use of a three-way stopcock for taking blood pressure in recovery room with blood pressure (anesthesia) cuffs.

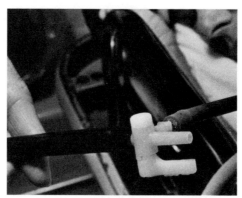

Figure 8-2

In the patients who have circulatory impairment, such as peripheral vascular disease, shock, and hypovolemia, it is often very difficult, if not impossible, to palpate pulses in the extremities or to measure systolic pressure by Korotkoff's sounds with the conventional stethoscope. A small oscillometer, the Doppler, is a valuable device to use in such situations.

Some helpful Pearls in the use of the Doppler to assess the peripheral pulses follow.

Pearl (6) Palpate Lightly

Place Doppler *lightly* or palpate lightly at the pulse location to prevent obliteration of the pulse from undue pressure.

Pearl (7) Anatomical Location of Pulse

Place the Doppler transducer at a peripheral pulse site (one of the grooves near bones where arterial pulsations are more easily detected).

Pearl (8) Detecting Blood Pressure

In order to check pressure (systolic only) the Doppler can be used along with an aneroid device (the pneumatic cuff with the sphygmomamometer). This is particularly useful when the stethoscope for the Korotkoff's sounds is highly unreliable (as in patients in shock). If you are checking the systolic pressure, locate the pulse with the Doppler, by inflating the cuff (which has been placed on the extremity) approximately 30 mm above the point on the gauge that the pulse was obliterated. Slowly (at approximately 3 mm/sec) deflate the cuff. Record systolic pressure at the reading the pulse is detected on the Doppler.

Pearl (9) Inexpensive Gels

You can save on the expense of using commercial gels for monitor and EKG leads by applying an inexpensive hair gel such as Dippity-Do—it works terrifically.

Pearl (10) Use of Finger-Cot

Using a Finger-Cot that is lubricated, digitally locate the anal orifice prior to the insertion of the thermometer, suppository, enema or rectal tube in those patients who cannot be turned on their side for adequate visualization of the anal orifice. This prevents unnecessary probing and subsequent trauma to the patient.

Pearl (11) Weighing the Patient with Bedscales

When the patient's condition does not permit him to be weighed out of bed, bedscales can be used.

Points to keep in mind in ascertaining accurate weight safely with minimal movements of the patient include:
1. When at all possible, plan this aspect of care in advance so that another person will be available to assist you with this procedure.
2. Use a lift sheet and an overhead trapeze bar to aid in moving the patient onto the weighing board.
3. Balance the scale first (recommend using a sheet or bath blanket and Chux if there is drainage or incontinence).
4. Make certain that the entire board is over the bed prior to placement of the patient on the board.

Pearl (12) The Flashlight Check for Worms

Small pinworms *(Oxyuris vermicularis)* often leave the rectum, particularly at night when the child is sleeping. They cause itching of the anus and may lead to other problems such as vaginitis. An older method of detecting the pinworms was by smearing the anus with shortening (lard). However, a simple flashlight test will help you detect them. When the child is sleeping, quickly shine the light at the anus, without disturbing the child, and observe for worms. They appear to be small white threadlike objects moving about the anal region and/or vulva.

Pearl (13) Inserting the "S"-Airway

Turning the patient on his side while mildly hyperextending his neck helps maintain a patent airway. Unfortunately, stretchers in the PARR are often much too narrow to accommodate this lateral positioning. Therefore, it often becomes necessary to insert an S-shaped oral airway. When inserting the airway, use the following maneuver (note Figure 8-3).

Insert the airway with one continuous smooth-sliding clockwise rotation (counterclockwise if you are left-handed). Note in Figure 8-4 the position changes of the proximal (internal) tip of the airway. Far too often, time and motion are wasted trying to insert the S-shaped airway with the incorrect method. With already many of the patients having compromised oxygenation, this waste of valuable time should be avoided.

Remember the patient's behavior usually provides cues for when this airway should be removed. The behavior may be gagging as he becomes more responsive, or he may actually cough it out as he becomes more alert.

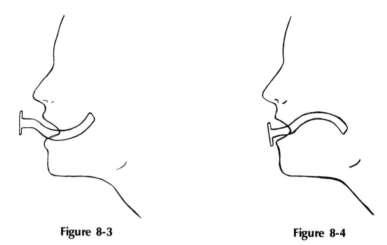

Figure 8-3   Figure 8-4

ASSESSMENT OF PHYSIOLOGICAL PARAMETERS

Pearl (14) The 6 P's Assessment

When checking the extremities for circulatory impairment, for example in a patient with peripheral vascular disease (PVD), the following code may serve as a reminder to include all of the major points to assess. Check for:

1. Pulselessness—no pulse
2. Pyrexia—temperature (fever)
3. Parasthesia—sensation (decreased)
4. Paralysis—movement (loss of)
5. Pallor—color
6. Pain—discomfort in the extremity, at rest or with activity

Pearl (15) X Marks the Site

For frequent pulse checks in peripheral vascular disease or after arteriogram or cardiac catheterization, mark the site where the pulse is felt the first time you find it. Then you will know where to look each succeeding time. Not only will you save time, but you will make the patient feel more secure by finding the pulse quickly and surely each time.

Pearl (16) Audible Cues for Assessing Respirations

To the nurse in the PARR assessing the respiratory status of the postoperative patient is a priority and requires the nurse's special senses. Some of the cues can be detected simply by *listening.*

1. Is there snoring? This often occurs due to the relaxation of the soft tissues with resultant partial blockage of the airway by the tongue and other soft tissues.
2. Is there a change in respiratory pattern?
3. Is there quiet where once there were audible breath sounds?
4. Are there gurgling or choking sounds?

   It is essential that the nurse stay alert to such sounds. Without *prompt* intervention, maintenance of an adequate airway may be lost. Also delay in reestablishment of a patent airway may require that the nurse and medical team resort to severe measures. (For instance, once laryngospasms occur, a tracheostomy or other drastic measures may be necessary rather than simple pharyngeal suctioning.)

Pearl (17) The Gag Reflex

Checking the return of the gag reflex is important in assessing progress in the postop patient. Be sure to use a 1) tongue depressor, 2) plastic bite-stick and 3) oral S-shaped airway instead of an applicator, your finger or a twist of gauze. The latter can result in injury to the patient or nurse and airway obstruction.

Pearl (18) Assessing a Groin—Temperature

When the temperature cannot be checked rectally or orally, particularly in your obese patients, an alternative to checking axillary temperature is to place the thermometer in the groin area. Hold the thermometer in place for five minutes. As well as being close to an ample blood supply, the thermometer can be placed in this area easily.

Pearl (19) Early Clues When Ambulating

Place your arm about the patient's waist when you are assisting him with ambulating. In addition to giving better support, you can detect early clues that he is becoming weak or is about to faint. Such clues include increasing warmth in the area, perspiring, and/or tightening of the muscles in his back.

Pearl (20) Is the Drainage CSF?

If you are watching a patient who has had a skull fracture or for some other reason could have a cerebrospinal fluid (CSF) leak, here is an easy test: If the patient has clear drainage from his nose or ear, dipstick the drainage for glucose. If the dipstick is positive, the drainage is probably CSF.

MONITORING LEADS TO INTERVENTIONS

Pearl (21) Descriptions of Transport Bed—SICU

Our staff members have found the transport bed most helpful. Note Figure 8-5 and the following instructions.
1. Have bed made to include hypothermia.
2. Plug the life pak monitor and suction machines into chargers (and be sure they are plugged into a wall outlet).
3. Have clean set-up for ventilator after each patient (call Resp. Therapy).
4. The O_2 tank should be at least at the 1,000 level at all times.
5. Cardiac arrest board should be in place under the draw sheet.
6. The following drugs should be on hand:
   a. Sodium bicarbonate
      1. Adult—1
      2. Pediatric—1
   b. Lidocaine—1
   c. Epinephrine 1:10,000—1
   d. Atropine—1
   e. Calcium chloride—1

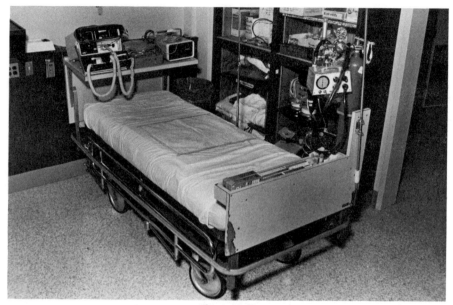

Figure 8-5

    f.   Bacteriostatic saline—1

    g.   5 cc syringe, 19 g needle—1

7.   Also on hand should be :

    a.   An airway of appropriate size.

    b.   Suction catheters of appropriate size.

8.   Operating room (OR) courier will come for bed when patient is to be transported postsurgery.

9.   Emergency transport from unit for x-rays, etc. should utilize bed.

10.   After the patient is settled, remove equipment from bed and replace regular footboard and headboard from another bed.

11.   Directions for use: life pak—inside of upper lid—read carefully. Check defibrillator two times per week.

12.   Procedure for use of portable suction:

    a.   Charge the power pack after each use. Charging time for discharged battery is 12 to 14 hours. Batteries are fully charged when the green light goes out. To avoid overloading, disconnect the charger a few hours after the green light goes out.

    b.   On-off switch—one step—low suction; two steps—high suction.

    c.   Water container should be filled with distilled water. It is used to clear the suction catheter and tubing after each use.

    d.   Vacuum bottle holds over one pint. When filled remove it, empty contents and cleanse with disinfectant.

    e.   To clean: all parts, except motor and power pack, are dismantled and cleaned in a disinfectant, hot soapy water, or, if necessary, by boiling.

    f.   No harm occurs if aspirated matter enters the pump. However, the pump will have to be dismantled and cleaned (see instruction book).

Pearl (22) Double-Made Surgical Transport Bed

Note the illustration in Figure 8-6. Cover the mattress with fitted sheet. Place the hypothermia blanket on the bed. Cover the hypothermia blanket with a bath blanket. Place a draw sheet over this. Two disposable drainage pads are positioned on the center of the bed and a cardiac arrest board is placed in the area of the bed where the patient's thorax would be. Then an additional bath blanket, draw sheet and drainage pads are added to the bed.

When the patient arrives from surgery, the top drainage pads, draw sheet, bath blanket and the arrest board are removed, which leaves a clean bed under your patient.

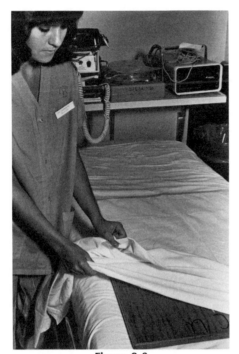

Figure 8-6

Pearl (23) Advantages of a Transport Bed

The advantages of the transport surgical bed include:
1. Provides rapid transport from the OR to the intensive care unit.
2. Eliminates need for excessive moves such as from OR table to stretcher, from stretcher to bed in SICU.
3. Aids in preventing alteration in vital signs from the sudden position changes which are encountered when the patient must be moved from bed to bed.
4. Saves valuable time from the need to change the bed soon after surgery. It allows the nurse to prepare this bed in advance.
5. Makes emergency drugs and supplies immediately available at bedside.

Pearl (24) When Baby Forgets to Breathe

We are all familiar with thumping baby's feet when his apneic monitor sounds, but here is a new thought. Nurses in the Neonatal Intensive Care Unit tie a piece of twill tape around the baby's ankle and then put it through the window of the isolette. If baby experiences apneabradycardia, a short quick tug on the tape will often stimulate him enough to continue breathing without having to open the isolette.

The following Pearls are for use when administering iced lavage.

Pearl (25) Isotonic Saline

When iced lavage is needed to aid in promoting hemostasis in patients with gastrointestinal (GI) bleeding, keep the lavage sterile and isotonic. A supply of sterile saline should be kept in a refrigerator for immediate use during an emergency.

Avoid pouring saline over a basin of ice. Why? As the ice melts, the solution is no longer isotonic nor sterile.

Pearl (26) Keeping the Solution Near

When possible, place an overbed table or bedside table draped with a Chux or towel near the patient. The patient can be more closely observed, there is less chance of dripping and spilling the saline on the floor and linen, and there is no wasted motion.

Pearl (27) Recording Intake-Output

Keep a record of the amount of irrigant used and the amount and description of the return.

Pearl (28) Necessary Supplies

Provide a large sterile wash basin in which to place the bottle of saline. Pour ice into the basin, around the saline bottle.

Provide a sterile irrigation tray containing a medium-sized basin, and a sterile asepto syringe. Also provide another *large wash basin and graduated container.* The return should be placed into the graduated container for measurement of output. The graduated container can be emptied into the large wash basin. This prevents halting the procedure to empty the graduated container.

Pearl (29) Assessing and Reassuring

Remember this patient is bleeding and may have abnormal vital signs or cardiovascular parameters. Be certain to help prevent the patient from becoming too hypothermic by checking vital signs frequently throughout the procedure, covering with blankets and noting the level of consciousness. Help allay fear and apprehension by reassuring the patient in a calm manner. One *can* work efficiently and rapidly without appearing rushed and disorganized.

Pearl (30) Effective Treatment of Beginning Sacral Skin Breakdown

Here is one helpful way to treat beginning decubitus ulcers of the sacrum (note Figure 8-7).

1. Place the patient on his or her abdomen.
2. Separate the gluteal fold, taping each buttock to one of the patient's siderails. Long strips of plastic drape (e.g., Steridrape) can be substituted for the tape.
3. Prep the area surrounding the decubitus and the decubitus ulcer itself with Betadine solution.
4. Apply Maalox to the decubitus and apply a heat lamp to the area for approximately 15 to 20 minutes, or until the Maalox is completely dry.
5. Repeat the procedure once or twice per shift until the area is healed.
6. Remember to use appropriate measures which promote privacy during this procedure.

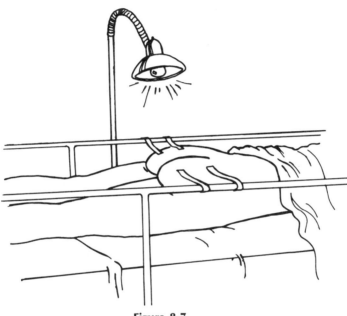

Figure 8-7

Infection control and safety

Chapter nine

Maintaining a safe and healthy environment is an important function of the nurse in promoting the optimum well-being of the patient. Improper use of equipment, failure to adhere to the principles of asepsis, prolonged use of catheters, and debilitating illness are just a few examples of the many factors which contribute to nosocomial (hospital-acquired) infections.

While communicable diseases and other infections exist, it is the nosocomial infections which you can often prevent. Improper lighting, faulty equipment, abuse and misuse of procedures, etc. infringe on the patient's safety.

The Pearls in this chapter focus on the following three main objectives which are essential to promoting a safe and healthy environment in caring for your patients:
1. To prevent and decrease the occurrence and transmission of infections.
2. To safeguard the patient from dangers in his environment.
3. To practice personal safety.

MAINTAINING ASEPTIC TECHNIQUE

Pearl (1) Double Gloving

Double gloving can promote sterility, save time and maintain safety (e.g., it allows one person to do tracheostomy care without having to stop and reglove). By double gloving for trach care, once the inner cannula has been removed for cleaning, the outer gloves can be quickly discarded and then you are free to continue cleaning of the inner cannula and completing the suctioning procedure. This helps decrease the patient apprehension by limiting the time involved in this procedure.

Pearl (2) The Sterile Field—In Dressing Changes

Occasionally improvising in a procedure to save supplies, time, and expense is often in disharmony with the sound basic principles of asepsis. Consequently, as procedures are altered for meeting the individual patient situations, it is essential that careful evaluation of these alterations is made. *Creativity and improvisations which are incorrect or unsafe are not one and the same.*

For example, in pouring a solution over gauze sponges which are in their sterile packages, unless this package is wax-coated or specially treated for moisture-proofing, contamination occurs (see Figure 9-1). The principle abused here is that moisture transfers organisms from unsterile surfaces (table top or bed, wherever package is lying) to sterile surfaces.

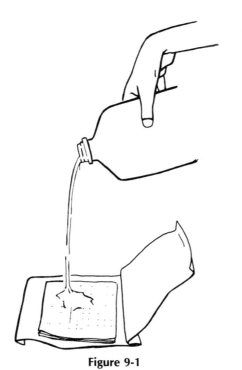

Figure 9-1

Another example is the needless practice of pouring small amounts of solution from a bottle before using the solution. One need only consider the length of time it takes to chemically render an object or surface sterile by soaking it in a potent disinfectant to realize this practice should be discouraged.

Pearl (3) Removing Soiled Gloves

With hand A grasp the cuff of B (opposite glove). Pull this glove off into glove A. Then with the *ungloved* hand, grasp the cuff of A glove and pull it off over the B glove, resulting in both gloves being inverted with the soiled sides inside (note Figure 9-2). Discard them into the waste container.

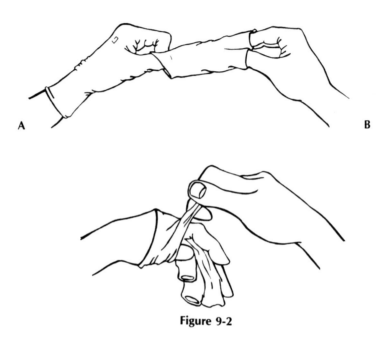

A   B

Figure 9-2

Pearl (4) Freeing the Glove Fingers

Need to reverse the glove? Are the fingers of the glove not fully extended? Need a right-handed glove and you only have a left-handed glove?
1. Invert glove inside itself as needed.
2. Hold glove at cuff.
3. Flip the glove over quickly several times toward you (until there is fullness or a ballooning effect).
4. Grasp cuff tightly with one hand to maintain the fullness by preventing air leakage.
5. With the free hand squeeze the glove from palm outwards. This extends ("pops" without tearing) the fingers free.
    This procedure should be used only when other gloves are not readily available and a delay would present problems.

Pearl (5) The Telltale Lines

Checking sterile-wrapped packages for expiration date, rips and tears, wetness, etc., in order to ensure the use of *sterile supplies* for patient care when needed is a common practice. However, one must also observe the autoclave tape to note if the markings (usually diagonal lines on the tape) have *darkened*. If this telltale sign is missing, the package has not been autoclaved, and the sterility must be questioned.

Pearl (6) When a Sterile Item Must Be Placed on a Sterile Field by a Nonsterile Person

Items should not be flipped onto a sterile field when they can be placed without contaminating the field. Flipping even a pack of sutures requires experience, and there is always the hazard of disrupting other items on the field. (See Figure 9-3 for *incorrect* method. Note the nurse's arms are over the field.)

Here is how to add a package of sterile gauze sponges to the field (Figure 9-4). Principle: No reaching over or across the sterile field with an unsterile hand or item.

Standing away from the field:

1. Grasp the edges of the package with thumbs and pull apart enough to open the package.
2. With one hand, place forefinger on the upper edge and the thumb immediately posterior (below the edge).
3. In an all-in-one movement pull the package open, while leaning *toward* (but not over) the field with the hand which is covered by the package.
4. The item is placed on the sterile field without the package wrapping touching the field.

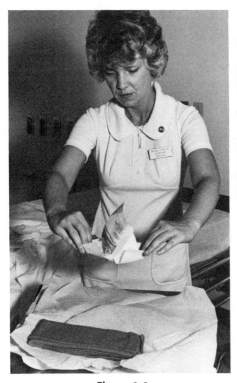 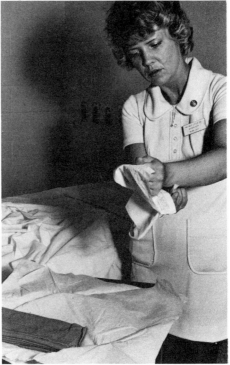

Figure 9-3   Figure 9-4

ISOLATION
Pearl (7) Isolation Guards

Post isolation signs on the patient's room door when needed. These signs should also cite the precautionary measures that should be followed by all entering that patient's room (use of gown, mask, or gloves only, etc.). Merely stating the type of isolation to be enforced is not adequate. These signs can be made by the staff. They are also supplied commercially (note Figure 9-5). Use of these signs helps facilitate continuity of infection control by staff and family members.

WOUND AND SKIN ISOLATION

VISITORS: Report to Nurses' Station before entering room!

Private Room: Desirable.

Gowns: Must be worn by all persons having direct contact with patient.

Masks: Not necessary except during dressing changes.

Hands: Must be washed with a Povidone Iodine Scrub on entering and leaving room, and after contact with excretions or secretions of the patient. (NOTE: HAND DE-GERMING IS THE SINGLE MOST IMPORTANT MEANS OF PREVENTING THE SPREAD OF INFECTION.)

Gloves: Must be worn by all persons having direct contact with infected area.

Articles: Special precautions necessary for instruments, dressings, and linen. *Dressings* should be handled with sterile surgical instruments. Used dressings should be placed in an impervious plastic bag, which can be closed securely, double-bagged, and incinerated without being opened.

Linen: Double bag in plastic inner bag with linen outer bag.

Figure 9-5

Pearl (8) Removing Nondisposable Dishes and Trays from Isolation Rooms

Ideally when a patient is placed on enteric isolation, it is best to use precautionary measures such as disposable food trays and dishes. However, when nondisposable trays and dishes are in the room, they should be removed to help facilitate a clean environment. This can be done by having a person stand outside the room door with a double-layered plastic bag (one bag placed inside the other) or a newspaper envelope.

How to prepare a newspaper envelope for collecting the tray and dishes:
1. Open four double newspaper pages.
2. Place pages evenly on top of each other.
3. Staple three sides securely.
4. Leave one long side open for receiving the dirty tray and dishes.

Another method of preparing a newspaper envelope (Figure 9-6) is to:
1. Open two double newspaper pages.
2. Place one opened Chux (plastic-lined) over the pages of newspaper and one below the newspaper.
3. Staple three sides, leaving one long side open, for placement of the dirty tray and dishes.

A supply of these isolation tray envelopes can be prepared in advance. Once the staff is ready to remove the tray from the room, one person in the room gathers the tray and slides it into the isolation-tray envelope which is held by someone outside the room door. Avoid contaminating the exterior parts of the bag or the receiver. Once the tray has been placed in the envelope, the open side is folded closed and secured by stapling. (Tag envelope with an "Isolation" sign.)

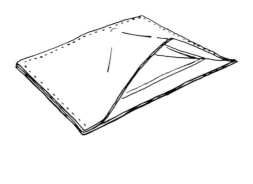

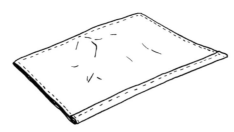

Figure 9-6

Pearl (9) Removing Contaminated Gown

When removing a contaminated gown, as you prepare to leave the isolation room, untie the bands at the waist and bring them around to the front of the gown, looping them to prevent their touching the floor.

Be sure to wash your hands thoroughly before reaching near your face to untie the neckband. After untying the neckbands, pull off the gown by grasping the cuffs. Then discard it into the appropriate hamper.

Pearl (10) How to Knot a Full Plastic Bag

Do you or your staff find it difficult to tie a plastic bag which is at the point of overflowing with trash or dirty linen, and there are no ties or rubber bands at your finger tips? Here is a method of tying your fullest plastic bag, *if* it can be tied at all.

1. Grasp the two sides together in the center of the bag opening.
2. Roll edge over at least one turn.
3. Grasp the two corners and pull together tightly from the outer edges of the bag and tie the corners into a "granny knot."

Tying this bag in this fashion will keep it closed securely.

RADIUM IMPLANTS

Pearl (11) Prevent the Patient from Being a Lonely Radiation Source

While the nurse modifies her nursing care plan to prevent unnecessary exposure to radiation from her patients who are receiving radioactive isotopes as treatment, it is essential that she provide appropriate interventions for dealing with the psychosocial needs of the patient as well as his principal needs. These patients often have complex psychosocial problems involving fear of the unknown, fear of prognosis, separation anxiety, pain, etc.

The nurse should organize care in order to have time to visit the patient and sit at a safe distance from the bedside. Much emotional support is provided for the patient by the nurse coming to his room at times when the administering of a treatment or performance of some task are not necessary. Such visits should be included as part of the plan of care. These can be accomplished without unnecessary exposure to radiation. Collaborate with the radiation therapist as to the precautions necessary.

Pearl (12) A Flexible Visitation Schedule

Plan with the family a flexible schedule for visits by the family and/or close friends. Since the length of time one person can be in the room is limited, such a schedule provides more satisfactory visitation and emotional support to the patient. Check with radiation therapy to see if a lead apron can be used to lengthen visits safely.

Pearl (13) Prevent Unnecessary Exposure to Radioactivity

When caring for patients who are temporarily radiation sources, special precautions are necessary for safety to the personnel caring for him as well as for the patient. If it becomes necessary to have two of the patients in the same room, it is essential that the bedside table, drainage bags, etc., all be placed on the outer extremes of the patient's bed. This prevents unnecessary exposure to the nurse. She can then avoid the need to work *between* two sources of radiation when caring for either of the patients. Three precautionary principles must be adhered to for safety: 1) time, 2) distance, and 3) shielding.

SAFETY WITH IV THERAPY

Pearl (14) Hang the Extra Tubing

You note the physician's orders advise you to encourage the patient to ambulate. The patient has an infusion. With a portable IV pole, a piece of tape and a paper clip he is set to go. You realize the excess length of IV tubing has many advantages but presents a problem for the patient who is ambulating. Therefore, where and how can the tubing be secured safely? Figure 9-7 illustrates the tubing secured by the following process.

1. Open a paper clip so that the clip resembles an "S."
2. Tape the S-shaped clip to the IV pole at a level below the patient's waste.
3. Place the extra length of the tubing in the lower hook of the "S."

The clip can remain in place for the patient's future walks. (Some of the recently developed infusion sets have a small plastic built-in handle which serves the same purpose as a paper clip.)

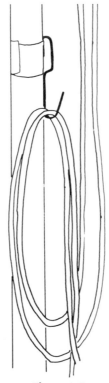

Figure 9-7

Pearl (15) Cover the Stopcock

Here is one way to keep an open end of a stopcock from being contaminated when it is not in use. Aseptically, remove the black rubber tip from the plunger inside a sterile 3 cc syringe. This fits nicely over the stopcock opening.

Pearl (16) Corking the Stopcock

Keep sterile corks to use as substitutes for the rubber tips of the stopcock when they are misplaced.

Pearl (17) Repairing the Stopcock

When the rubber tip on the stopcock is displaced, the tip of a 3 cc syringe works well and safely in its place. This eliminates the need to replace the entire stopcock, thus avoiding unnecessary expense.

Pearl (18) Storing the Rubber Stopcock Tips

Save the rubber tips, which are removed from the stopcocks as needed. Place these tips in a jar of antiseptic solution, such as 1:1000 aqueous zepharin or alcohol.

SAFETY IN THE OPERATING ROOM
Pearl (19) Defogging the Spectacles

What an annoyance to discover that one's spectacles are fogging a short time after donning a mask! To solve this problem, simply 1) wash the glasses in soapy water; 2) do *not* rinse; 3) wipe dry; and 4) place the edges of the mask under the brim of the frames.

Pearl (20) A Drop of Water for Dry Soles

In operating suites where explosive agents are used and the need for conduction is important, a conductivity device is used. The nurse steps on the device to check conductivity of shoes, booties, etc.

For those staff members who fail to register within the safety range on this device, the problem may be due to the lack of perspiration (or dry soles). Place a drop of water inside the shoe on the sole of the foot; then recheck for conductivity.

Pearl (21) Those Flying Strays

1. Using a wet prep solution and a wet towel as you shave the patient in the operating room will prevent the straying of loose hair.
2. Use the sticky side of adhesive tape to gather the loose hair when a dry prep is used.

Pearl (22) No Extra Sponges to Miscount

All sponges which are used for prepping should be removed from the operating room before the surgery begins. These are removed along with the used prep tray and kick-bucket. This provides a cleaner environment and can prevent incorrect sponge counts should these sponges accidently be included in the count.

Pearl (23) Contaminated OR Cases

Place a towel saturated with disinfectant (e.g., amphyl) as a doormat outside the operating room that has a "contaminated case." This, along with the other precautionary measures which are being used, will aid in preventing the spread of infection.

Pearl (24) Sterile Light Handles

To save time and provide for ease in focusing the over-the-table light in the OR to the operative field, use light handles which are autoclaved. With these handles, the surgeon can adjust the light exactly where it is needed (note Figure 9-8).

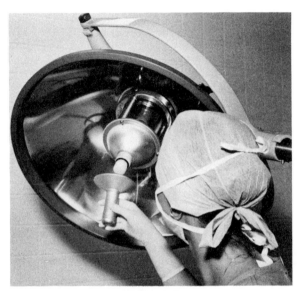

Figure 9-8

SAFETY IN THE USE OF CASTS AND PLASTER OF PARIS

Caring for patients in casts or assisting in applying a cast requires an understanding and some experience in dealing with plaster of paris. We anticipate that you will find these Pearls helpful.

Pearl (25) Special Cast—Care Cart

For areas in which casts are more commonly applied, prepare a special cart equipped for this purpose. This cart can be brought quickly into the room. In the small hospital emergency room or on the orthopedic unit, it may be kept in a special "cast room."

Pearl (26) Protective Covers

Protect bed, tables, floor, etc. from plaster by covering them with sheets of plastic or newspaper. Dried plaster is very difficult to remove.

Pearl (27) Note Cues for Pace

When applying the cast, do not prepare several rolls of plaster of paris in advance, as they will often dry before the doctor is ready to use them. Observe and assist at the physician's pace.

Pearl (28) Exothermic Reaction

Dip the rolls of plaster into buckets of water which are about room temperature (70° F). Plaster of paris produces an exothermic reaction. If warmer water is used, it will become too hot and you will also lose some of the plaster from the roll unnecessarily as it begins to set too rapidly.

Pearl (29) Passing the Roll

Do not wring the roll of plaster but smooth it gently before handing it to the doctor.

Pearl (30) Clogged Drain

Do not empty the plaster pan into the lavatory unless a special plaster trap has been installed. It may clog the drain.

Pearl (31) No Finger Indentations Please

Hold the cast with your palms until it is dried.

Pearl (32) Assessing the Patient with a Cast

When caring for the patient who has a dried cast:
1. Feel the cast for "hot" spots, which may indicate infection.
2. Use your sense of smell, particularly for a musty odor—this also could mean an infection.
3. Remember the boy who called "wolf"—patients who are immobilized to some extent as with casts frequently complain of discomfort, boredom, etc. Always investigate these complaints; you may save a "limb and a life."
4. Assess for adequate circulation.

OTHER SAFETY MEASURES
Pearl (33) Padding the Rails

For the toddler who must be on bedrest, it sometimes becomes necessary to pad the siderails to prevent the restless child from injury. Be sure to leave the holes between the slats open. This is necessary to prevent sensory deprivation.

Pearl (34) Bandaging with Ace Wrap

1. Place the patient in a comfortable position, supporting the part that is to be bandaged.
2. Use good body mechanics, and get yourself into a comfortable position to apply the bandage.
3. Never allow two skin surfaces to remain in contact as bandaged. Place Telfa strips, gauze pledgets or absorbent cotton between skin surfaces as needed (between the toes, under the breasts, padding under arms or body prominences).
4. Always hold the roll of bandage uppermost (see Figure 9-9).
5. Apply the bandage beginning distally on an extremity and moving it toward the trunk. (Note Figure 9-9 for correct wrapping.)
6. Unwind the bandage as you apply it (avoid unwinding extra bandage in advance).

7. Secure the bandage initially by making *two circular turns* around the extremity.
8. When possible, leave the digits exposed to observe for adequate circulation.
9. With each turn of the bandage, overlap the area just applied by one-half.
10. Avoid making extra turns to use all the bandage. This makes the pressure uneven, causing discomfort.
11. Do not leave gaps or skin surfaces exposed to conserve on the amount of bandage used. (Note in Figure 9-10 an *incorrect* wrapping.)
12. Question your patient about how comfortable the bandage is.
13. Inspect periodically for tightness, etc., and instruct the patient to notify you of any numbness or discomfort.

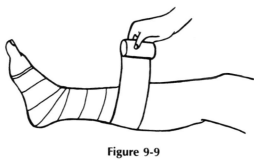

Figure 9-9

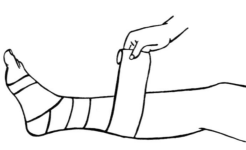

Figure 9-10

Pearl (35) Should the Electric Power Fail

In the event of power failure, certain equipment must be checked *immediately*. Compile and post a list of the equipment to check in such an emergency. Company representatives can furnish details about their equipment in event of power failure. Two examples which require the nurse's attention in order to ensure patient safety are:

1. Mechanical respirators—patients must be removed and ventilated manually.

2. Electrical suction pumps—the patient with water-sealed chest drainage attached to electrical suction devices must have the tube to the suction control bottle disconnected to allow for adequate ventilation and prevention of a tension pneumothorax.

Pearl (36) Seizure Precautions

Keep a padded tongue depressor at the bedside (note Figure 9-11). Cover the tongue depressor with a gauze sponge and wrap securely with tape. Cover the *entire* blade with tape, so that a portion of the tape can be grasped in your hand to prevent a potential airway obstruction from dislodgment of tape from the blade as it is moistened by the saliva.

When a patient is having a seizure, do not attempt to restrain him, this only aggravates the contractions and you may be injured. Pad the rails or use pillows during the tonic-clonic convulsions of the seizure to prevent the patient from injury.

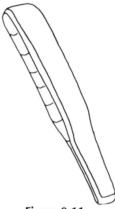

Figure 9-11

Pearl (37) Stats and Tourniquet at Bedside

Keep a hemostat and a tourniquet taped to the head of the patient's bed as a precautionary measure, should hemorrhage occur from the stump site of the amputee.

CLEANLINESS OF THE PATIENT AND ENVIRONMENT
Pearl (38) Help the Patient Control His Environment with a Trash Bag

The patient on bedrest who is awake and alert can become frustrated with his lack of control of his surroundings. If he happens also to be a patient who uses a large number of Kleenex (such as a tracheostomy patient or an oral surgery patient) or for some other reason seems to create a lot of small trash, place a waste receptacle within his reach. Simply tape a small plastic, foil-lined or waxed bag (open) to the siderail of the bed. He will appreciate not having to look for the waste basket and not having a messy bed or overbed table.

Pearl (39) Wet and Dries

Include Wet and Dries at the bedside or recommend that a supply of these be available for purchase in the giftshop or on the volunteer "store on wheels." These are particularly well-received by the in-bed patient.

Pearl (40) Personal Hygiene Kit

Set up a supply of admission kits. These are given to the patients. This kit should include small toilet articles (toothpaste, Kleenex, lotion, etc.).

Pearl (41) That Dirty Gomco

Before disconnecting the Gomco or other suction machine, turn on the suction and run water through the tubing and into the suction receptacle. This maintains better care of the equipment and prevents unnecessary work for someone else after the mucus, blood and other drainage have dried in the equipment.

GADGETS FOR INFECTION CONTROL AND SAFETY

Pearl (42) Recycling Broken IV Poles in the Patient's Bathroom

The top part of a broken telescoping IV pole can be taped to the vertical safety bar in the patient's bathroom to provide a convenient place to hang the patient's IV solutions while he uses the bathroom. This is especially useful in two cases.
1. The patient who is able to care for himself and would appreciate a moment's privacy.
2. The patient who is weak or poorly coordinated who would be likely to fall. (Hanging the IV bottle gives the nurse two free hands.)
       This is also better than hanging the solutions on the back of the door because IV tubing is less likely to be tripped over or tangled and because the tubing will not be pulled by the sudden opening of the door.

Pearl (43) A Paper Cup Funnel

Cut the bottom from a Dixie paper cup and place it in the neck of the hot water bottle or ice bag. This cup acts as a funnel and makes filling the container much simpler and faster.

Pearl (44) Temporary Moisture to Trach

Until a trach nebulizer arrives, use a moistened four-by-four gauze square to place over tracheostomy. This should be 1) sterile; 2) replaced frequently; and 3) large enough, porous enough and *without a cotton filler* to prevent occluding the tracheal opening.

Pearl (45) Soap the Diaper Pin

If you will stick the sharp edge of a safety pin into a bar of soap prior to pinning the diaper, the pin will pass through the diaper easier. This helps prevent bending and breaking of the pin as well as sore hands if you are pinning many diapers throughout the day. (Always prevent accidental sticking of the infant with the pin by placing your hand between baby and the diaper when pinning.)

Pearl (46) Use of Double Suction Adaptor

When the patient situation demands the use of more than one suction apparatus at the bedside (such as for sumps and tracheal suctioning), you can eliminate the need to use an extra portable suction machine at the bedside by the use of the double-suction adaptor which fits in the wall suction outlet. Eliminating unnecessary equipment prevents an unsafe, cluttered environment (note Figure 9-12).

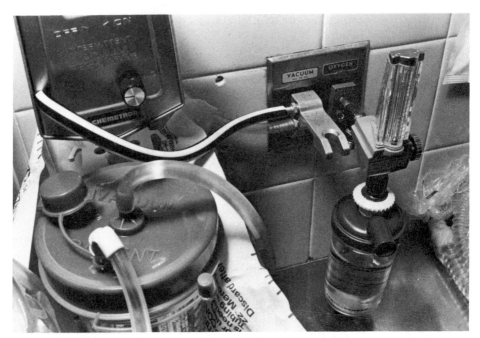

Figure 9-12

Pearl (47) The Aqua-Pad—Safe Heating Device

Hot water bottles and heating pads should only be applied when there is a doctor's order, particularly on the patient who is sensitive to temperature changes (such as patients with parasthesia, peripheral vascular disease, and the elderly patient). Of the heating devices, the Aqua-Pad which is electrically controlled is one of the safest. Since the temperature is regulated by a key which is preset by the staff, the patient does not have access to the key, and the danger of his altering the temperature control causing burns is eliminated.

Pearl (48) Prepackaged Glove

For a simpler technique and a better asepsis when suctioning the patient, use a prepackaged glove-suction catheter (note Figure 9-13).

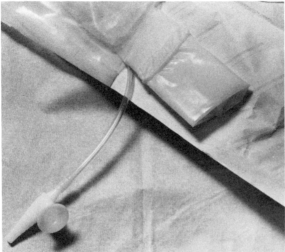

Figure 9-13

Pearl (49) Tying Restraints to Siderails

Tying restraints to movable rails is hazardous and should be avoided. (Note Figure 9-14 for a correct placement of restraints. They are secured to the bed and not to the rails.)

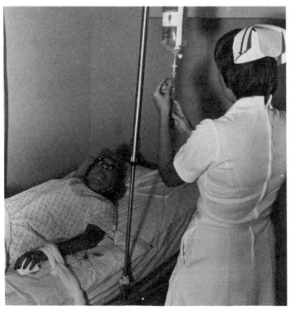

Figure 9-14

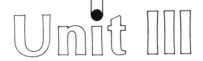

Pearls for
nursing
management

Unit III

Management in the clinical setting

Chapter ten

Effective management in the clinical setting involves the coordination of the services provided by the members of the health teams. This requires team support, effort and cooperation from *all* of the staff to provide for continuity of quality patient care.

As the nurse, you must recognize your responsibility as the key facilitator in establishing and maintaining a rewarding and organized environment in order to achieve those goals which provide quality health care.

Too often the problems of inadequate health care, disorganized nursing units, job dissatisfaction, etc., are directly related to poor management. This can range from lack of planning and inadequate assignments to not keeping necessary supplies available on the unit.

Of these problems, a major factor which contributes to this inadequate management and implementation of patient care is *poor communication* with others.

This chapter offers Pearls that can be applied to promote quality health care through appropriate management, which can be adapted to your particular clinical setting. Specific considerations dealt with are the nursing report, nursing rounds, written documents, care plans, organizing supplies, communicative techniques, and inservice education, among others.

It seems appropriate for the first Pearl in this chapter to be the "Nurse's Motto" contributed by Frances Daniels, a nursing assistant on the neurosurgery wing.

Pearl (1) Nurse's Motto

"Put yourself in your patients' place; treat them as you would like to be treated." Not a bad way to treat staff members either.

STOCKING THE UNIT, REQUESTING SUPPLIES, AND LOCATING EQUIPMENT

Next we have nine Pearls involving stocking the unit, requesting supplies, and keeping track of equipment belonging to the unit. No one enjoys working on a poorly stocked unit, and much time can be saved by keeping supplies where they can be found. Therefore, tips like these have a direct bearing on the day-to-day life of the unit.

Pearl (2) Checking Supplies

It is essential for a well-stocked, organized unit to devise a system of delegating responsibility for checking and ordering stock supplies. This can be done in conjunction with other departments (e.g., housekeeping, central supply) by the supervisor, head nurse, or delegated to another nurse or the unit manager.

Pearl (3) A Clipboard for Requesting Supplies

Regardless of what system is used in keeping supplies in stock on the unit or how this responsibility is delegated, you will find it helpful to include this tip.

Place a clipboard at a convenient location so that staff can list a gadget, device, dressing, etc. which is needed as they perform their assignments. This saves time and facilitates the stocking of supplies when used along with the routine stock list.

Pearl (4) Post Lists, Lists, Lists

To save time when trying to find a piece of equipment or a medication, it is helpful to provide lists with which one can note at a glance the location of what he is looking for.

For example, on your large supply carts attach a list (enclosed in plastic envelope to prevent soiling, so that it can be removed for changes and read at a glance) of supplies and what shelf they are on. Another example is to post three-by-five cards on the front of cabinet drawers listing medications or supplies in the drawers.

Pearl (5) Organize with Supply Cart

A well-stocked supply cart (similar to the commonly used isolation cart) placed outside the patient's door aids the nurse in organizing patient care more effectively for those who are receiving radioactive isotope treatment.

Pearl (6) Make a Choice

On each of our CSS carts we have hung a sign that instructs the nurses to "make a choice," comparing the contents of three sizes of dressing trays, emphasizing the *time* spent assembling these materials without using the tray (see Figure 10-1). This serves three purposes:

1. It reminds the nurses of the contents of the dressing trays.
2. It is a reminder that time is spent by assembling dressing materials and could be saved by the use of a dressing tray.
3. It is a quick note that says, "Whatever you are getting, save time and get it all in one trip."

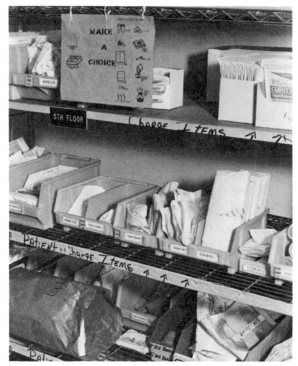

Figure 10-1

Pearl (7) Clear the Dumbwaiter

If your hospital has a dumbwaiter service to central supply room (CSR), use it efficiently. Avoid unnecessary delays in removing the ordered piece of equipment, dressing, etc.

Should the tray, dressing, etc., arrive but no longer be needed, inform the staff in CSR of this by returning the tray with an attached cancellation slip or by returning the tray and notifying the CSR by phone or "wall squawk box" on the unit (by which messages can be received in CSR). This aids in:

1. Better communication between staff in CSR and on the patient units.
2. Eliminating misplaced or "lost" equipment.
3. Preventing unnecessary charges and expense to your unit.
4. Providing room on the dumbwaiter to send other equipment.
5. Eliminating extra phone calls.
6. Saving the staff's time on both the nursing unit and in CSR.

Pearl (8) Is the CSR Request Complete?

If the request which is sent to CSR is a stat request, be certain to mark it accordingly. Also, be sure to stamp the unit location from which the stat request is sent. Otherwise, you may find yourself in for a long wait and an unfilled stat request.

Pearl (9) Reporting of Faulty Equipment

Remove from the patient's room, when possible, equipment which needs repair. Report all malfunctioning equipment, electrical shocks, frayed wires, etc., to correct departments. Label equipment which is not operating correctly and set it aside when possible.

Pearl (10) Properly Labeled "Return to X Location"

Avoid misplaced property and cluttered rooms by labeling equipment trays, etc., using indelible ink. State station number and label "Please return to 'X'" (nurse's station, clean utility room, etc.).

BECOMING FAMILIAR WITH THE NEW UNIT, EQUIPMENT, PROCEDURES AND POLICIES

Pearl (11) The Multi-Varied Bedrail "Gizmos"

How many times have nurses been delayed in administering care to the patient by having to stop and search for that "gizmo" (latch, button, etc.) that allows one to lower the siderails? With so many different types of hospital beds, it is important for the nurse to become as familiar with the basic operation of the patient's bed as she does with the other equipment involved in assuring safety, comfort and immediate care. Include this detail as part of orientation to new units or hospitals, etc.

Pearl (12) Becoming Familiar with the New

When adopting new procedures, materials, etc., it is often very helpful to provide a simple display on the staff bulletin board or table in the coffee-conference room where the staff will have more access to it.

Pearl (13) The New Gadget—A Blessing or a Headache?

How many times have you found yourself attempting to use a new piece of equipment which seems totally impractical and certainly less efficient than the old one which was "carted away"? Such a situation can be prevented by:

1. The nursing staff being represented on the committee responsible for selection and approval of new equipment and supplies which involve nursing care.
2. Asking that representatives from the various companies provide appropriate lectures, instruction manuals and even demonstrations of their gadgets while identifying the advantages and disadvantages.
3. Providing an adequate inservice to the staff members as needed. This might involve simply sharing brochures on the unit or laboratory sessions where a demonstration and practice in use of the equipment is necessary. (For instance, the staff's rejection of new equipment or misuse and abuse of the equipment often stems from lack of familiarity with its mechanics.)
4. An occasional window-shopping—a visit to the local or nearby surgical supply store can provide an excellent opportunity to become acquainted with a tremendous variety of useful gadgets and supplies which are available for patient care.
5. Providing suggestion boxes for various recommendations and complaints that deal with supplies and equipment.

6. Promoting creativity of the staff by recognition of the most valuable ideas submitted for improving patient care, saving time or cost, etc.

This should involve all of the hospital personnel. For instance, in some hospital systems a recognition awards ceremony is held annually to recognize the creative ideas contributed by the personnel. This stimulates healthy competition among the staff as well as producing valuable results for the hospital. Example: one of the hospital cooks submitted a diagram of a gadget which was a terrifically efficient cost-time saver in cooking a particular breakfast food.

Pearl (14) The Treasure Hunt

To orient newcomers to your unit, try a treasure hunt. We have found this helpful in 1) breaking the ice as they become acquainted with the staff, and 2) orienting them to the surroundings of that particular unit.

The treasure hunt can be adapted to meet the particular situation. For instance, when you are orienting no more than two new staff members you may choose to instruct each newcomer to find a staff member, be able to identify his name and position and inquire of this staff member where the emergency cart is located or other such information.

With a larger group such as a group of student nurses beginning their clinical experience on the unit, a three-by-five note card can be given to each student with instructions such as:

"If Mr. Jones in Room 201 was complaining of pain and requesting his analgesic, identify *each step* in the *process* of determining if an analgesic can be administered:
a. establishing *if* an analgesic is ordered;
b. if it is time to be given;
c. procedure for signing out the narcotic;
d. location of narcotics, and medication cup or syringe; and
e. on what sheet the medication would be charted as having been given."

It is helpful to set a time limit for the treasure hunt and have the students report back to the conference room to share their findings with the group. Each student would be given a different "treasure" to find.

Pearl (15) Four Tips for the Observer in the Operating Room

Occasionally, the observer in the operating room becomes ill, weak or may actually faint. This can cause problems such as a) the minor distraction of needing assistance from others in the room, b) contamination of the sterile field, or c) injury of the observer from falling, should he lose consciousness.

To help prevent this situation, the following measures should be emphasized (particularly to newcomers in the surgical suite):

1. Eat breakfast (if early case) or a carbohydrate snack, prior to coming to the suite. Occasionally the weakness is simply due to hypoglycemia.

2. Shift body weight when observing. The observer often depends on others to show him where to stand, either on a small step stool or in a certain area for better observation. While the newcomer must limit mobility to prevent contamination to a sterile field or disturbance of the team, he should be encouraged to shift his weight from one leg to another, and to avoid folding his arms or standing in such a rigid position that his circulation is hampered.

3.   Arrive early enough to practice wearing the mask before observing the surgery. For the observer who may be unaccustomed to wearing the mask, there is a tendency to hyperventilate or feel like he is smothering at first.

4.   The observer should step back from the table, sit down, or leave the room immediately, should he become ill or feel faint. The nurse should watch the observer fairly often to detect early clues of his needing assistance.

Despite all the measures used to prevent the observer from experiencing these problems, they still may occur because of fear or anxiety, producing high-level stress from the actual observation of the surgical intervention, or from any combination of these factors.

PROMOTING ORGANIZATION

Next are eight Pearls dealing with the organization of that written information about the unit which needs to be at each employee's fingertips.

Pearl (16) The PARR Care Plan Card File

Keep a small file box of three-by-five cards (or a "flip-type" Kardex file) or "routine postoperative care plans" (postcoronary by-pass, post-TURP [transurethral prostatectomy], postspinal anesthesia, etc.). While modifications in actual care will be made to meet the individual patient's situation, the written established routines are very helpful in assembling equipment in advance, organizing daily assignments, evaluating the care, and providing a source of information for the newcomer in the postanesthesia recovery room (PARR).

Pearl (17) Card File for Diagnostic Tests

Keep a small three-by-five card file box at the nurse's station. Label the box "Diagnostic Tests." List the preparations which a patient will need for the test (e.g., for a liver biopsy the nurse would note that a type and match for a unit of blood, a liver biopsy tray, and a permit to be signed may all be required in that particular hospital or on that particular unit. Examples of other tests include lumbar puncture, IVP, barium enema, gall bladder series, etc.). Though tests and preparation for tests may be modified to meet the individual needs, these established routines save time, promote continuity of care, and help prevent omissions in the preparation.

This box is often referred to by the nurse and the unit clerk, as the orders are being transcribed from the chart and treatment cards or Kardex are being prepared.

Pearl (18) Kardex for Diagnostic Procedures and Tests

This file will include a Kardex on each test commonly used on that unit or in that hospital. Each Kardex card should include the following information:
1.   Purpose of the test
2.   Brief description of the procedure
3.   Special care following the test
4.   The major complications, or side effects
5.   Recommended therapy for complications (This is necessary in order to have necessary supplies on hand should the need arise.)

Pearl (19) Using a Patient Location Board

To make bed assignments, to answer relatives' questions, to check on equipment, and for a multiplicity of other reasons, the nurse and the clerk often need to know *quickly* which patient is in each room. Here is how this need is met:
1. Make a schematic diagram of the patient rooms and beds on your unit.
2. Label the room numbers and the bed spaces.
3. Cover this with plexiglass.
4. Now write patient's names with a wax pencil on the plexiglass.
We use the following code system:

> Red = male patients
> Blue = famale patients
> Black = patients who are being admitted but are not here yet

Also, if a patient is being discharged, his name is underlined with a solid line. If he is being transferred, his name is underlined with a broken line. Further patient requests (such as a private room) and alerts (such as "two Smiths—Abel 579, Baker 581") are written in black wax pencil.

Pearl (20) A Patient Movement Board

The ambulant wing has involvement with 22 services of attending physicians, chief residents, residents, interns, and medical students, as well as having students of other disciplines on the unit. There are constant requests by family members to know where patients are and what time they left the unit. To always be organized and on top of patient movement (and to free the nurse or clerk from constantly having to look up the information), this board was designed:

PATIENT MOVEMENT BOARD

X-Ray procedures   *Surgery*
Jane Doe   RFL   Pat Jones   Obesity By-pass
Time out _____   Time out _____

Joe Brown   Cysto
Time out _____

Mae Webb   UGI   ~~CANCELLED~~

Pearl (21) A Patient Treatment Board

The treatment board meets the need for immediate, *correct* information on each patient on the busy ambulant wing. As the night nurses check charts, they make a list of all treatments, preop, etc., and place the information on the treatment board, which is a bulletin board arranged as follows:

PATIENT TREATMENT BOARD

24 Hour Urines	S&A's 30 min ā C qid
321 A J. Thomas	
322 B M. Jones	Needs Transportation
330 B B. White	320 A J. Jones w/c
Save Urine and Sputum	320 B M. Stable St.
319 A P. Black	Blind Patients
318 B J. Birch	
	NPO
Intake and Output	
325 A M. Peterson	Special Diets
Force Fluids	

It is a chalkboard and is placed so that it is visible to everyone in the nursing station. The medication nurse is responsible for keeping the board updated. It is an efficient and accurate time-saver as it makes clerks and nursing assistants easily aware of the special needs of all the patients and able to relay this information to the appropriate people without having to call the nurse. Headings are on colored paper. Patient names are on white.

The treatment board lends itself to any type of treatment. It is *now* information kept updated by the team leaders each shift. This is especially helpful in an area like the ambulant wing, where patients are off the unit much of the day for x-rays, procedures, minor surgery, etc.

Pearl (22) A Weight Record Worksheet

When it is necessary to assess weights for a large number of patients, prepare a weight record worksheet and keep it on a clipboard. Include a list of patients, days of the week, and method of weighing. Color-code by underlining the appropriate patient's block on the worksheet to signify the method of weighing needed (e.g., blue = weighs self; green = portable bathroom scales to bedside; red = bedscales).

Routine weights, either daily, once per week or every other day, are usually taken and recorded at 6 or 7 A.M. (which is usually before the day shift and breakfast).

Pearl (23) Clipboards for Data Worksheets

Hang clipboards on hooks at a convenient location near the chart rack in the nurses' station. Use the clipboards for ease in recording frequently needed data such as TPR's, weights, pressures, etc. Among the advantages of using these handy clipboards for such worksheets are the following:

1.   The accessibility to staff for recording or referring the data when charts are in use, such as when charts are being used by the medical staff on rounds, or the nurse is recording team medications.

2.   A quick source of information without having to pull individual patients'

charts from the rack (e.g., when information is needed on several patients at one time by the nursing supervisor, dietitian, therapist, physician, etc.).

3.   When transferring such data to charts is the responsibility of one person (e.g., unit clerk, head nurse, etc.; especially useful when functional assignments are used).

4.   Prevents duplication of data collection in many instances. It is important to remember to cross off the data on these clipboards (without obliterating it) once it has been transferred to the permanent record. This eliminates the wasted time of someone else pulling the charts to transfer data that has already been charted.

COMMUNICATION AMONG PEOPLE IN THE HOSPITAL

Visitors are a very welcome part of the life of a nursing unit, but there must be some way of controlling the length of their stay to ensure patient rest and well-being and to perform nursing care measures. Here is a lovely little Pearl dealing with just this.

Pearl (24) Limiting Visitors

1.   A quick dimming of light and/or soft-spoken but firm and polite announcement over the intercom is often all that is needed to announce that visiting hours are over.

2.   Visitor passes, which are distributed and returned to the volunteer or employee at a desk near the elevators or in the front lobby, aid in limiting the number of visitors at any one time.

Such systems provide more effective communication and foster better nurse-patient-family-visitor interactions. This often prevents the nursing staff or families or patients from having to ask visitors to leave.

Here is a Pearl that facilitates interdisciplinary communication in the care of the preoperative patient.

Pearl (25) A Preop Tool

To enhance communication among all the staff, patients and families who are involved in surgical visits (pre- and postop) devise a protocol and procedure which involves verbal input and written data. One such tool is the *checklist* as described: Establish a standardized preop visit checklist with space for additional comments, to individualize the care.

a.   Certain items on the checklist are initiated by the staff on a patient's unit and any additional comments are noted. This is kept in a Kardex or on a clipboard on the patient unit near the surgery schedule so it is readily available to others.

b.   As the anesthesiologist, surgeon, patient service representative visits with similar checklists, they add to and select data from this checklist.

And here is a Pearl that facilitates the coordination of the sending and receiving unit when a patient is transferred.

Pearl (26) The Timely Transfer

When transferring patients from one unit to another (e.g., recovery room back to patient's own room), consider the following helpful hints for a smoother, safer transfer:

1. Avoid transferring patients during staff mealtimes. (There are often a limited number of staff on the units during this time and there will be less assistance available.)

2. Avoid transferring patients during changes of shifts.

3. Notify the unit to which the patient is to be transferred *in advance* so better preparations can be made for receiving the patient (e.g., they may need to order additional equipment, move beds in order to place this patient closer to the nursing unit, or call for an orderly to assist in the transfer).

Here are six Pearls that deal with effective communication between groups of people in the hospital setting.

Pearl (27) Routine Care Plans

While the plan of care must certainly be individualized for each patient situation, it is most helpful, particularly for staff members who are not familiar with a particular unit (the new employee, the staff nurse who is relieving during vacation or illness from another unit, etc.), to have a Kardex or card file of the routine care for the particular type of patient, for example, a card file for patients who have transurethral resection (TUR's), the patient who has received a spinal, or the routine care plan for mothers who are breast feeding.

These must be stated concisely and simply. If they are to serve a useful purpose, you must include only the major points of care in terms of priority. It is also essential that you stress to the staff using these routine plans that they only serve as an organizational guide and in no way eliminate the need for judgment and decision making in providing and planning individualized care for each patient.

Pearl (28) Discharge Criteria

Have you ever found yourself confronted with the following situations?

a. Asking the patient to postpone leaving for home with his family until you have had a chance to collaborate further with the medical staff, therapist, dietitian, etc., regarding his discharge.

b. Questioning whether the patient should be discharged, even though the order was written to do so, due to a change in the patient's condition.

Some of the indecisions and last minute postponements can be avoided by the nursing unit having access to prepared *discharge criteria* for its patients. Many factors must be considered. A few points are: 1) At what point in his rehabilitation can the orthopedic patient who has had "above the knee amputation" be discharged? 2) What physiological parameters must be met (e.g., temperature—afebrile for 24 hours? 72 hours?)?

This planning and formulation of appropriate discharge criteria involves the health team. The nurse is often the one who must initiate and coordinate the process.

Pearl (29) Print a Booklet about Your Unit

Printing charges are really not very high if you print in large quantities, especially if your hospital has a printing center. Several of the individual units at Shands have printed booklets describing their units. The booklets are given to patients (especially elective admissions) and their families.

Examples of things to include in such a publication are:

1. The purpose of the unit.
2. An explanation of the surroundings.
3. A description of the personnel (why they wear scrub suits, why they wear masks, what levels of personnel there are, how do you tell them apart).
4. An explanation of isolation procedures (use drawings).
5. An explanation of visiting hours.

The booklet should be relatively simple, colorful, and as nonthreatening as possible, and it should convey an attitude of warmth and caring to help put the family and/or patient at ease. Our families have especially appreciated the realization by the nurses that they want to know these things. The nurses have appreciated being able to inform families even when they do not have time to talk at length, and knowing that the patient and family have something *in writing* to refresh their memories if they are too anxious to comprehend what they hear.

Pearl (30) The Patient and Family Speak Out

Provide a checklist or simple evaluation form for the patient and/or his family to complete prior to or upon discharge. This can be placed in a suggestion box located in the lobby or, if the patient prefers, he can return it by mail.

Pearl (31) The Chart Cover Signals

Use chart covers which have a device that signals others, drawing their attention to the chart. Some chart covers can be purchased with such a device. Others must be improvised by the unit staff.

The device may be designed in a variety of ways and serve specific functions. The overall function of these devices is to serve as a mode of communication. Examples include:

1. A flap which can be turned down that extends beyond the chart cover edge. (This may be color-coded to indicate a specific message such as a message to the doctor from the nurse-dietitian therapist.)

2. Two flaps, color-coded—one indicating there is a new order on the chart, and another indicating stat order (this one is usually coded red) which communicates to the staff to pull this chart first when transcribing orders from the chart.

3. A slot near the top of the chart cover. With a slide of a button, the slot is opened. When the slot is open, this signals a preestablished message (e.g., "Doctor, the medications need updating"). Once the message has been received the slot is pushed closed.

These devices should certainly never be used to replace direct communication and interaction with others, but they can facilitate the communication system. Advantages of such a device are:

1. Permanent devices are more stable and more likely to get a message to another person than sticking notes on chart covers.

2.   They save time and often prevent the need for additional phone calls should the nurse be involved in patient care when the health team member is on the unit, or if the health team member can be on the unit for only a brief visit on that particular occasion.

Pearl (32) Standard Abbreviations

While certain abbreviations are commonly used in most hospitals and health agencies throughout the country, each hospital or health agency should compile a list of accepted standard abbreviations to be used in charting for that particular facility. The list should be readily available and kept near the charting area.

For certain areas, an additional supplemental list should be prepared (e.g., in certain specialty areas such as dialysis, coronary care, and GYN clinic inclusion of a supplemental listing of terms peculiar to that area is helpful).

Use of a compiled list of standard abbreviations facilitates clearer communication in charting and prevents errors due to lack of clarity.

NURSING ROUNDS

Here are some Pearls about getting new ideas from the staff and giving new information to the staff. Often the latter takes the form of orientation.

Pearl (33) On Soliciting Opinions

When soliciting written opinions or suggestions from your staff, you will find that you have a better response if you will include the following measures:
1.   Provide a *closed* suggestion box or suggest that each individual submit his packet of written suggestions in a sealed envelope.
2.   Meet with the staff in advance and explain the purpose; offer an opportunity for questions and comments.
3.   Give a deadline for returning their responses.
4.   Post a reminder on a bulletin board in a strategic location (e.g., coffee room).
5.   Praise the group for their contributions as they are returning.
6.   When appropriate, be a contributor yourself to start the ball rolling.

Pearl (34) The Communication Book

When it is beneficial for staff members to be able to communicate directly to the entire staff, including the supervisor, use a "Communication Book." An inexpensive composition book works well for this. A bound one is better than one with rings, since pages are less likely to fall out of a bound composition book.

The book can be used to express suggestions, complaints, thanks, new ideas, welcomes for new staff members, goodbyes to and from old ones, wedding and birth announcements and congratulations, and party invitations. Surely there are other uses as well. Entries may be signed or anonymous. It is helpful for those who read each entry to initial the margin to indicate that they are aware of its contents.

Supervisors can use the book for announcements and reminders, thereby getting a message quickly to the entire staff.

Too often nursing rounds border on a monotonous routine. Here are eight suggestions you will find helpful in keeping rounds meaningful and effective for all involved (staff and patients).

Pearl (35) Consise Report

Give a brief concise report on a few patients (three to six), then make rounds on these patients. Repeat the process until you and the staff have made rounds on all the patients on your designated team or unit. This method permits more attention to the individual patient as the staff correlates the correct information shared in the report with the specific patients on rounds because the focus is limited to only a few patients. Also, since the staff is not sitting in a distant conference room but standing a short distance from the patient's room which they are about to enter, there are other favorable effects, such as: the reports becomes more concise, avoiding lengthy overtures; the staff are less likely to sit and doze until it is time to make walking rounds; and time is saved and repetition avoided. This eliminates a lengthy report of all the patients followed by the grand tour of walking rounds.

Pearl (36) Introductions—Please!

Introduce the patient to the group, and particularly single out the staff member who is assigned to care for him.

Pearl (37) Put Your Presence to Best Use

The effects of your tone of voice, eye contact, touch, etc., when applied appropriately with a pertinent statement that makes the group see the patient as an individual, cannot be underestimated. For example, avoid this *poor approach:* The nurse leader barely glances or nods her head in the patient's direction, and focuses on her worksheet or looks only at the staff and remarks, "This patient is OK, nothing significant in his care, just the routine. Won't need to make his bed as he is being discharged this morning.") Use a *good approach*, such as: Walk over and use direct eye contact, as you talk with the patient, "Mr. Jones, I'm Ms. Elliott, the team leader, and this is the staff who will be on duty this shift. Mr. Thomas will be caring for you today." (Give Mr. Thomas and Mr. Jones a moment to exchange comments.) Make to the staff and particularly to Mr. Thomas such comments as, "Mr. Jones had a problem with headaches for a couple of days after surgery, but these stopped yesterday." "How are you feeling now Mr. Jones?" "The physician wrote a discharge note last evening. Did he discuss this with you?" "So your wife is coming for you at 10 o'clock this morning. Well, we are glad to see that you've made such progress in your recovery." "Mr. Thomas, will you assist Mr. Jones in getting ready for discharge? Also, feel free to keep me posted if I can be of assistance to you, Mr. Jones or Mrs. Jones when she arrives, in answering any particular questions."

Pearl (38) Bedside Assessment

Assess the patient and his needs, checking equipment, dressings, etc., but avoid focusing strictly on the gadgets and neglecting the patient.

Pearl (39) Let's Hear It from the Patient

Ask the patient for input. The nurse leader or the staff member assigned to care for the patient should jot a reminder on her work pad in front of the patient as the patient makes a request, etc. This serves to reassure the patient that his needs will be noted and keeps the staff from forgetting to follow through on the comments or requests.

Pearl (40) Events for the Day

Also, use nursing rounds as a time to make certain that the patient is informed of his plan of care for the shift (for example, he is due at x-ray about midmorning or his physical therapy appointment is cancelled for this morning).

Pearl (41) Spontaneous Teaching

Nursing rounds is a time to note pertinent feedback from the patient, in order to teach and intervene more appropriately then and later, for example, "I've misplaced my glasses," or "Do you know a friend told me he had bad headaches after his spinal anesthesia?"

Pearl (42) A Role Model

The nurse leader sets an example of role model. Often the way you relate to your patients will influence how your staff interacts with them. Nursing rounds should be included as an integral part of the day's activities. The rounds can be modified to fit the needs of the particular situation or setting (e.g., adult versus pediatric units; small rural hospital versus large metropolitan hospital; limited staff versus plentiful staff; chronic versus acutely ill patients; large open wards versus individual rooms).

THE NURSING REPORT

Pearl (43) The Conference Room Report

The disadvantages of having the staff sit in the conference room for a report on all the patients were discussed. The *advantages* include:
1. There is more privacy.
2. The staff is less likely to be interrupted than when reporting as you make rounds.
3. Occasionally it saves time.
4. Once the staff is assembled in the conference room, assignments and other activities can be handled during the session, either preceeding or following the report.
5. When there is limited staffing, it aids the staff who is going off duty, as they complete last minute tasks and answer call lights, to contact the group receiving the report and the nurse leader who is giving the report.

Nursing reports take time both to give and to receive. They should be an essential mode of effective communication between shifts to provide continuity of patient care on a 24-hour basis. The specific type of report and the technique used in sharing it will need to be modified to best meet the needs of that particular unit.
Several modifications may include:

Pearl (44) A Taped Report

This is prepared by the nurse who is reporting off duty. It will require organizing a concise orderly report. Also, it will require setting aside a time interval (usually 10 to 15 minutes) to tape the report near the end of the shift. Keep notes on your worksheet or note pad in an orderly fashion throughout the shift. This will save time later when trying to tape the report and prevent omission of pertinent facts.

The taped report frees the nurse reporting off to complete her charting, etc. while the next shift is hearing the report. However, this nurse must be sure to:
1. Be available should there be questions.
2. Report any new changes in patient status at the conclusion of the tape, as necessary.

The staff who is listening to the tape should feel free to stop the tape when necessary. Though interruptions should be kept to a minimum, questions and comments may best be discussed for clarity by stopping the tape, rather than waiting until the tape is concluded. The head nurse should use her discretion and judgment regarding this.

Pearl (45) The Team Report

When there is more than one team on the unit, it is only necessary for team members to receive the report for their patients. While it would save time to have reports being given to the respective teams, simultaneously, the lack of space and/or staffing often prevents this. Consequently, while the first team is receiving a report, the other team can use the time for brief team conferences, problem-solving, staff enrichment, updating care plans, reviewing the latest data on charts, gathering supplies for treatments, etc.

PERSONNEL SUPERVISION

Here are five Pearls that deal directly with personnel supervision.

Pearl (46) Keep Track of Employee Attendance

To keep track of attendance systematically, use a blank monthly time sheet for each employee. List the months down the left side, the dates across the top. Each month when the schedules are posted, print the employee's days off on his schedule. When he calls in sick, is absent or late, write this also on his schedule. At the end of the year, at evaluation time, you will have a complete record of each employee's attendance for the year.

19___																		NAME			
	1	2	3	4	5	6	7	8	9	10	11	12	13	14	15	16	17	18 . . .			
Jan.																					
Feb.																					
March																					
April																					
May																					
June																					
July																					
August																					
Sept.																					
Oct.																					
Nov.																					
Dec.																					

Pearl (47) Who Are You?

Throughout the hospital and on each nursing unit, proper identification of others is important. Staff must wear name tags. (Should a name tag become lost or left at home, improvise one from a piece of tape and place on the uniform.)

Teach your staff, and establish the habit yourself of asking "Who are you?" of those visitors or staff who do not have proper identification.

Pearl (48) For Managing Employees

Give maximum assignment at beginning of shift—never add to anyone's load, but take away by doing some work for them. This helps build rapport and improves morale.

Pearl (49) Praise-Reprimand

When dealing with staff, administrators (head nurse, etc.) should remember to praise in public and correct or reprimand in private.

Pearl (50) Don't Ignore First Symptoms of Poor Performance

Some good advice in the form of a Pearl: It does not save hurt feelings, it does not make things go smoother, and it does not save time or energy to let poor performance go unnoticed. Unchecked, it will probably get worse and worse until something has to be done. At this stage the corrective measures will be much more extensive and the employee much more devastated. More likely than not he will say, "Why didn't you tell me sooner?"

To put it more graphically, the first symptom of poor employee performance should not be ignored any more than should the first drop of pus from a wound.

GADGETS AND A LIST OF HELPFUL RESOURCES

Following are some Pearls dealing with little gadgets that can be used in managing the clinical environment.

Pearl (51) Stop the Walking Books

Need the PDR? dictionary? hospital formulary, etc.? For various and sundry reasons, ward (unit) libraries soon become depleted, leaving the staff in need of valuable sources of information. To aid in keeping the books on the unit, chain them to bolts in the wall near a desk where the staff can easily locate and use them. (The chains should be long enough so that the staff can sit at the desk or stand and use the books comfortably.)

Pearl (52) Metal Hanger Becomes a Clamp

The metal hanger which is supplied now by some companies to hang the infusion bottle at a lower level when more than one infusion is flowing can be twisted and used as a clamp (to hold the control switch and call light device at the bedside within easy reach of the patient).

Pearl (53) Special Racks

It is helpful to have a rack placed on the wall outside of the patient's room door. A clipboard containing patient history, record of vital signs, laboratory slips, any part of the patient's record can be placed in these racks. This is particularly helpful in the clinics where there are many patients.

When graphics and flow sheets are placed in such racks, they should be reversed to prevent visitors walking by the room from reading other patients' records (note Figure 10-2).

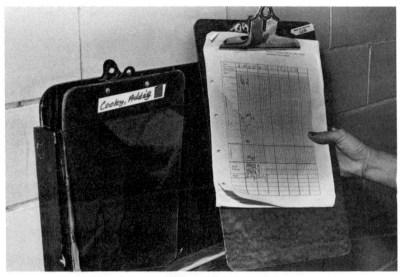

Figure 10-2

Pearl (54) Three-Ring Notebooks for Bulky Charts

A common three-ring notebook can be used as a chart binder, preventing the frustrating "fall out" of papers with the spring binder when a chart gets bulky (Figure 10-3).

Various forms of chart racks accommodate notebooks: a stationary circular rack at the nursing station and a rack that looks like a rolling bookcase (Figure 10-3) are examples. The rolling bookcase is especially useful because it can be taken on rounds or to the conference rooms.

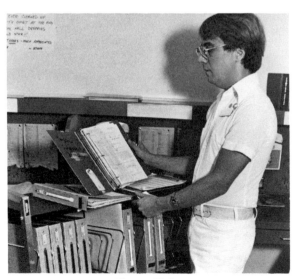

Figure 10-3

Pearl (55) Placement of Chart Tables in ICU

By placing overbed tables at the foot of the beds in intensive care, and providing adaptable stools, the nurse can observe the patient while charting. However, this is not designed for a limitation of the nurse's mobility away from the bedside. Without a greater mobility in the room, while providing adequate observations, the nurse would be more apt to experience sensory deprivation and greater level of stress (Figure 10-4).

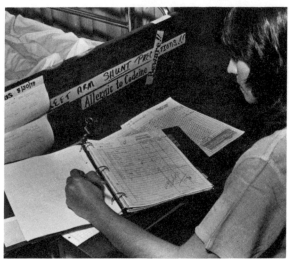

Figure 10-4

Pearl (56) The Tape Alert

1.   Place a piece of tape across the doorway whenever a special procedure is being performed (e.g., dressing changes in the burn unit). This is to notify others that they should not enter without knocking to be admitted by staff in the room and being properly attired, etc.

2.   Stretching a piece of tape across the floor in the operating suite serves as a reminder to staff and others that beyond this point measures in promoting asepsis are particularly important (masks up over nose and mouth, conductive booties on, etc.).

Pearl (57) Potty Training

Figure 10-5 depicts a helpful teaching tool used by our nursing inservice education staff in sharing helpful facts and simple instructions. The information is changed several times each week. The plexiglass holder prevents soiling. Examples of information shared varies and includes such items as "How to Convert Farenheit to Centigrade"; "Know Your Cleaners"; "Neurological Eye Checks"; etc.

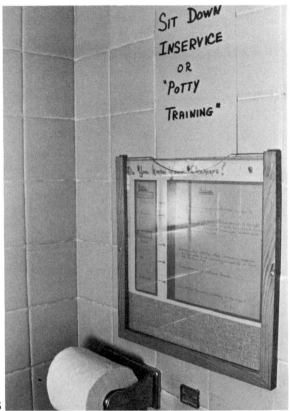

Figure 10-5

Pearl (58) Communicative Aids at the Bedside

Several bedside communicative aids which save time and often eliminate errors in treatment include the following:

1. Placing a wire rack over the foot of the bed for placing flow sheets. This permits immediate recording of data (vital signs, intake-output, etc.). It also provides the nurse and other members of the health team with a quick source of information about the patient's current status.

2. Place small slotted plastic plaques, which can be purchased commercially and installed easily at the bedside. Prepared messages can be slipped into these slots to convey reminders and information to others, such as: NPO; I-O; neuro checks, bedrest. Such messages can prevent errors which can be harmful or can prolong the hospital stay. For instance, the visitor may feel he is being helpful when he gives the patient who is NPO for surgery a glass of water. However, the nursing staff must keep this data current. Otherwise the information becomes incorrect and the staff will tend to disregard these as effective communication aids.

3. Placing a cork-type bulletin board (approximately two feet in height, one foot in width) can serve the same purposes as the previously cited aid. In addition, other messages or diagrams (e.g., for necessary position changes of the patient) or cheerful drawings by the child can be placed on these handy bulletin boards.

And here are some other resources:

Pearl (59) The Yellow Pages When Improvising Fails

When the local hospital does not have a gadget or helpful aid that would be very beneficial in patient care, improvise. When improvising is too time-consuming, or unsatisfactory in the particular case, ask the person responsible for ordering the supplies to check the yellow pages of the telephone directory for the nearest surgical supply company.

Pearl (60) Nurses' Drug Alert

This publication is helpful in providing information about current medication therapy. Compile the issues of this publication in a three-ring looseleaf notebook and place it in the nurse's station or other readily accessible area (e.g., conference or coffee room, or at the chart desk). It provides a handy and helpful drug information resource for the nursing staff. (*Nurses' Drug Alert* is published by Nurses' Drug Alert, Inc., 12 East 63rd Street, New York, N.Y., 10021.)

Pearl (61) Articles Relevant to Your Unit

Invite members of your staff to share articles from professional periodicals that are especially relevant to your unit. These articles can be collected in a looseleaf notebook or a file folder and made available to all interested employees. If you have physicians of several different specialties with patients on your unit, you may choose to have several notebooks, with one for each service.

Pearl (62) How About Nursing Consults

Something we have found useful is a list of nurses with clinical experience in different areas, such as oncology, pediatrics, neurosurgery, orthopedics, etc. By posting a copy of this list on each unit, with the names and unit phone numbers of expert nurses, we can more efficiently use the clinical knowledge of the working staff nurses.

Another way to do this is to provide the assistant director of nursing with such a list and have people from different units call her for a nursing consultation. This might be more effective if a fee were to be charged for the service.

Pearl (63) Use Your Community Agencies

Here is a hint that is especially good if you are moving to a new area or working in a hospital that does not have a public health referral nurse. Spend some time one day locating the local office of such agencies as the American Heart Association, the Cancer Society, the Lung Association, etc. and see, a) what services they can provide, and b) what their qualifications are for assistance to patients.

By doing this you may also find organizations that are *not* national but have developed specifically to meet a need in your community. Be sure to contact area churches; they may be very anxious to help families in distress while their family member is hospitalized, or to help with home care after discharge.

Here are some examples of some nationally known organizations. The list is by no means exhaustive:

Abortion Clinics and Counseling
Alcoholics Anonymous, Alanon, and Alateen
American Association of Retired Persons
The American Cancer Society
American Civil Liberties Union
American Foundation for the Blind
American Heart Association (Remember that they also have educational and other
        materials for vascular problems and stroke.)
Area Clinics for Indigent Patients
Area Drug Abuse Programs
Area Rape Counseling Services
Area Suicide and Crisis Intervention Service
The Arthritis Foundation
Big Brother—Big Sister
Bureau of Blind Services
Bureau of Workman's Compensation
Bus Schedules (from area and national transit companies)
Children's Medical Services
Communicable Disease Center in Atlanta
Diabetic Club
Easter Seal Society
Epilepsy Foundation
Family Planning Projects
Food Stamp Program
Foster Grandparents
International Association of Laryngectomies
Job Corps
March of Dimes
Meals of Wheels
Migrant Workers' Clinics
The National Kidney Foundation
Red Cross
RSVP (Retired Senior Volunteer Program)
Salvation Army
Social Security Administration
Speech and Hearing Clinics
United Way
Veteran's Administration
Vocational Rehabilitation
Your Civilian or Red Cross Regional Blood Center
Your Detail Man (Drug and hospital equipment companies often provide helpful
        pamphlets such as: Smith Kline and French, *Pocket Book of Medical
        Tables;* Ethicon, *Suture Use Manual: Use and Handling of Sutures and
        Needles;* Pfizer, *How to Give an Intramuscular Injection;* Hollister, *Stoma
        Measuring Card.)*
Your State Department of Health and Rehabilitation
Your State Mental Health Association

Many of these organizations have publications and audiovisual aids which could be very helpful for those providing programs for inservice education. Here are some examples of those available from the Cancer Society:

"Cancer Quackery"

"Educational Materials and Films for Nurses"

"How to Examine Your Breasts"

"Reach to Recovery"

"Rehabilitating Laryngectomies"

"Stay Healthy: Learn about Uterine Cancer"

"What Is Chemotherapy?"

There are many others, and most large associations have indexes of their publications which they can provide.

After making your calls and finding your information, compile it in an orderly fashion with a table of contents and make it available to the nurses in your hospital.

Health education

Chapter eleven

Promotion of health education is becoming an increasingly important part of the services to be provided for the consumer of health care by the various health care agencies. Whether you are preparing discharge criteria, organizing and planning staff development classes, or teaching the individual patient at the bedside, you should find the Pearls of the health teaching process described in this chapter beneficial.

Patient teaching is an integral part of the nurse's ever-expanding role and is an important part of her responsibility in promoting health education.

Pearls dealing with content or what to teach are interspersed throughout the book. However, health education involves much more than a) recognizing that it is one's responsibility to teach the patient, b) being knowledgeable of the content to be taught, and c) identifying the patients (clients) who need teaching.

In this chapter a major emphasis is on the process or the "how to teach" the patient and his family in order to achieve the best results. If the nurse can identify the process which occurs in this interaction with patients, families, or staff with whom she is involved in health teaching, then more precise modifications can be made as the teaching plan is evaluated.

With an awareness that an orderly process exists, the nurse should have a clearer perspective on the teaching role involved in health care. You will find that the Pearls that Ms. Joyce Stechmiller, the author-contributor of this chapter, shares with you focus on the following aspects of this process of health teaching:

1. Why are you teaching the patient (purposes, goals)?
2. What is compliance?
3. What are the factors that influence predictability of the outcome? How do you identify these factors?
4. What is the cost effectiveness of the nurse's, patient's and family's roles?
5. What should be involved in the role transition in patient teaching?
6. Was the teaching effective? How do you evaluate effectiveness?

The specific examples, case presentations, and the bibliography should prove helpful as guides for applying these Pearls as you teach in your specific health care setting.

It is the nurse's role and responsibility to institute effective health education when delivering not only secondary but also primary and tertiary care. The ultimate goal of the educational process is to change behaviors which will enable individuals to participate as active health consumers aimed at helping them recover from illness and maintaining health. This role would foster these behaviors: 1) self-triage with minor problems; 2) participation in systematic preventative care; 3) recognition of warning signs; and 4) commitment to the prescribed regimen. These health behaviors will be the focus of this chapter as well as factors that affect health behaviors. For example, nurses are striving to enable their patients to achieve specific health behaviors, including taking medications, following diets, decreasing delay in seeking care, keeping clinic appointments, and modifying risk factors, which correspond with the prescribed therapy.

The term used to identify the above behaviors is compliance. This word may rouse negative thoughts of patient passiveness. However, it will be used in this instance to not only describe the extent to which the individual understands his illness or risk of illness and adherence to medical instruction, but also to describe the degree of success in enabling this individual to be an active participant and decision maker in determining his health status.

Let us begin with a definition of health education. It is a *process* that bridges the gap between health information, the *content* or what you teach and the health *practice* (what the patient actually does). The teaching-learning process is dynamic, and in order to achieve behavioral change it demands constant planned interaction between the teacher and the learner, motivation, as well as the appropriate content material. The quality of the interaction seems to play a major role in this process. This is due to the fact that the learning process is dependent on the learner's perception of the teacher. Does the teacher believe in what he is teaching? Does the learner care about the learning situation? Is the learner satisfied with the relationship? Learning is internally controlled by the learner, not the teacher, engaging the whole being of the participant not only intellectually but also socially and psychologically. The learner needs support through praise and reinforcement from his family and friends perceiving their acceptance if he engages in the prescribed regimen. He must also be psychologically ready to participate, accepting of the illness or risk of illness. Individuals are motivated to learn if they see a need and perceive a personal goal that learning will help them achieve perhaps an asymptomatic state or a longer lease on life. They may invest their energy and change their behavior if they perceive their illness or symptoms of illness as severe enough. The key is to involve the learner and family using the principle of ego involvement which states that every individual tends to be committed to what he or she has participated in, making it a shared responsibility. If one simply imposes knowledge upon another, the result will be apathy, resistance, resentment, noncompliance and withdrawal.

The following are four valuable steps for an effective teaching-learning situation (see Figure 11-1).
1. Diagnosis of the individual's learning needs, through assessment.
2. Assisting the individual in discovering his learning needs to establish short- and long-term goals.
3. Selecting appropriate educational strategies for goal attainment.
4. Evaluation of educational goal attainment.

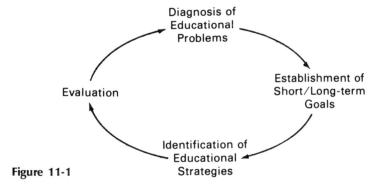

Figure 11-1

Diagnosis of Educational Problems

Establishment of Short/Long-term Goals

Identification of Educational Strategies

Evaluation

Step 1. Diagnosis through assessment

Clinical examples of this step (diagnosis of individual learning needs) are cited in Table 11-1 as follows:

	Table 11-1. Diagnosed Educational Problems	
HEALTH PROBLEM	**EDUCATIONAL PROBLEM**	**EDUCATIONAL OUTCOME**
1. Myocardial infarction (MI)	The patient does not believe that quitting smoking will affect his risk factor of another MI (perception of vulnerability-cost benefit)	To quit smoking
2. Uncontrolled hypertension	The patient does not take his medication because he believes it has caused impotency, but is unaware of the risk of stroke (perception of cost benefit and severity-vulnerability)	To take antihypertensive medications consistently
3. Congestive heart failure (CHF)	The wife refuses to prepare low sodium meals because she has always cooked with salt and does not understand how salt affects her husband's swollen ankles	To adhere to a 4 g sodium diet
4. Diabetes	The patient refuses to come back to clinic because he usually has to wait 2 to 3 hours to be seen by the doctor	To keep clinic appointments
5. Anticoagulation	The patient stopped returning to the clinic because he couldn't miss any more time from his job. Clinic only meets from 9 to 5, Monday through Friday	To return to clinic for weekly *prothrombin* times
6. MI	The patient does not understand how his getting out of bed and walking in the hall can affect his heart	To limit activities in the coronary care unit (CCU)
7. MI	"I don't know what I'm supposed to do when I go home. What medications will I have to take? When do I take them? Will I be able to take them appropriately?"	To take new medications following discharge from the hospital effectively

COLLECTING SUBJECTIVE DATA

To determine the learner's ability to participate in the learning process, it is important to consider the learner's understanding and perceptions which can provide necessary information in diagnosis of the individual's educational needs. When using the problem-oriented record format, the subjective data include the things the patient tells you. The following subjective categories can be assessed as determinants for predicting compliance and diagnosing educational needs.

Pearl (1) Perceptions of Illness and Risks

The individual's readiness to learn is greatly influenced by how he perceives his illness and the risks involved. Before jumping head-on into teaching the patient or others some valuable fact or procedure, explore the following in assessing his perception of illness.

1. *Symptoms of illness* (onset, duration, precipitating factors, alleviating factors, delay time and proposed therapy). For instance, why did the patient seek medical care in the first place? What does he think caused him to become ill? What can he do, if anything, to cause the symptoms to go away?
2. *Knowledge of proposed therapy.* What do I do? Why should I do what they tell me to do? How do I do what I am supposed to do? Will I be successful?
3. *Severity of illness or risk of severity.* How bad is my illness or risk? How do symptoms restrict my functional level? How does therapy affect severity?
4. *Vulnerability to illness* or recurrence of illness. How does therapy affect susceptibility to symptoms, risk of illness, illness?
5. *Cost benefit of prescribed therapy* to the therapy. What will happen if I participate with the prescribed therapy? Is it easier, more important, worthwhile, satisfying for me to participate with the prescribed therapy? Will it help me live longer? Will it alleviate symptoms?

Pearl (2) Prior Health Behaviors

Assessing the patient's prior preventative health behaviors will cue you in planning a realistic approach in the teaching plan.

1. What were his former patterns of administering prescribed medications? (knowledge of action, rationale, administration times, side effects, how often actually taken, why taken, and, if not taken, perception of consequences)
2. How has he used the health care system previously? (for systematic screening, for symptoms)
3. What has been his experience with health providers? (satisfaction, dissatisfaction)
4. What was his prior experience in the identification of symptoms and/or illness? (beneficial, nonbeneficial)
5. What was his prior identification of risk factors and need for modification?
6. What prior attempts were made to modify risk factors and success rates?

Pearl (3) Perception of His Support Systems

Who is the most important person to the patient? Does he think that his family or friends will help him with his therapy? Will they share his beliefs for therapy? Will they accept him more or less or the same if he participates with the therapy?

Pearl (4) Activity Level

Briefly describe the patient's typical weekday, including work status, weekend, habits, routines and norms. (Note Figure 11-2 for a summary of the preceding Pearls regarding subjective data.)

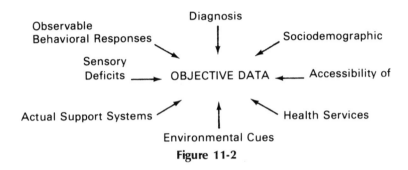

Figure 11-2

COLLECTING OBJECTIVE DATA

The objective findings are things that you observe within the learner's environment that will affect his health behavior and ultimately his educational diagnosis. The following objective data categories serve as important Pearls to be assessed when diagnosing the education problem.

Clinical examples of diagnosed educational problems were cited in Table 11-1, page 203.

Pearl (5) Actual Medical Diagnosis

What is the patient's medical problem, risk factors? Therapy and rationale: What does he have to do and why does he have to do it?

Pearl (6) Accessible, Available Health Services

Available health services include the health education plan, time and money available to teach, available staff, convenience to the learner, transportation and financial constraints.

Pearl (7) Actual Family-Staff-Social Support

Do the family, friends, and staff assist the learner through praise and reinforcement with the prescribed therapy, promoting compliance? Is there caring?

Pearl (8) Environmental Cues, Aids

Does the environment provide the patient with cues for recommended health behaviors?

Pearl (9) Sociodemographic Data

These data include the following:
1. Education level (reading, writing)
2. Language barriers

3. Ethnic background
4. Family structure
5. Health insurance
6. Financial status
7. Occupation

Pearl (10) Sensory Deficits

Sensory deficits may involve:

1. Attention span
2. Memory loss
3. Hearing defects
4. Visual disturbances

Pearl (11) Observed Behavioral Response to Illness

Note Figure 11-3 for a summary of the above Pearls dealing with objective data.

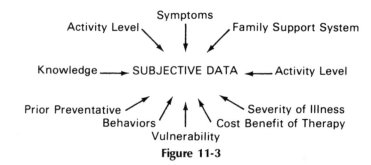

Symptoms

Activity Level   Family Support System

Knowledge ⟶ SUBJECTIVE DATA ⟵ Activity Level

Prior Preventative   Severity of Illness
Behaviors   Cost Benefit of Therapy
Vulnerability

Figure 11-3

STATING OBJECTIVES

Step 2.   Assisting the individual in discovering his learning needs is necessary to establish short- and long-term goals. Clinical examples of this step (assisting with learning needs) are cited in Table 11-2, page 207.

Pearl (12) Stating Objectives

To assist the individual to discover his learning needs and set short- and long-term educational goals, one should state objectives in terms of the desired change in health behavior. Ask yourself, what is it that the learner must do? What does he need to know in order to change the behavior? And what procedures and materials will work best to teach what I wish to teach? An objective is actually a desired educational outcome, describing the product of what a learner is supposed to be like, stating a proposed change in him, or a pattern of behavior or performance we want the learner to demonstrate. It is important for educational objectives to be identified because they provide structure and organization to your teaching plan, improve communication of the plan to the learner, staff and family, provide for continuity by the interdisciplinary team, and, finally and most important, provide a means for evaluating the teachers' and learners' efforts through statement of a performance, condition and criteria for evaluation.

Table 11-2. Clinical Examples of Assisting with Learning Needs

HEALTH PROBLEM	EDUCATIONAL PROBLEM	EDUCATIONAL OBJECTIVE
1. Hypertension	Not taking medication at home consistently because does not know the rationale and cost benefit	The patient will be able to take his anti-hypertension medication at home with 100 percent accuracy. The patient will know why he is to take his hypertensive medication by stating rationale and risk of hypertension with 100 percent accuracy
2. Potential atelectasis as a postoperative complication	Not performing breathing exercise because he has not been taught to do them	To perform deep breathing and coughing every 3 hours per day with 100 percent effectiveness as evidenced by clear breath sounds. To know that deep breathing exercises are necessary to prevent atelectasis by stating its importance
3. Continual diuretic therapy for congestive heart failure	Taking medications only when symptoms of uneasy breathing occur	To take diuretics as prescribed with 100 percent accuracy. To know by stating that diuretic therapy is necessary during the asymptomatic phase to reduce blood volume and extra work on the heart

How do you state an objective? First, identify the described behavior by name: for example, to take medications, lose weight, or quit smoking. You must specify the behavior that will be evidence that the learner has achieved the objective. Next, try to define the behavior by describing the condition under which the behavior will be expected to occur. For example, when requested, the patient will state the warning signs of heart attack. Finally, one must specify the criterion of acceptable performance by describing how well the individual must perform the activity, that is 100 percent of the time. For example, the patient will take his pulse prior to taking Inderal with 100 percent accuracy.

Now review this educational outcome. It divides a broad objective into its parts, identifying the sequences of a health educational goal. Consider the series of steps as short-term goals for the patient in taking his Inderal as prescribed with 100 percent accuracy.

1. Identifies medication by name, color, pill.
2. Can state administration times, dosage.
3. Can state the rationale for taking the medication.
4. Can state the side effects of the medication.
5. Can state the contraindications of the medication.
6. Can solve problems. What to do if the pills run out, if predefined side effects occur.
7. Knows what the consequences are if the medication is not taken.
8. Keeps log of administration times and pulse.

Toward this goal the individual should be assisted in discovering his learning needs and seen as a partner in decision making. He should have access to all information that is meaningful and he has a right to disagree with the teacher. In other words, he is an active participant in defining his educational objectives. This concept is the idea of the contract, which removes the traditional paternalism of the teacher, restriction of information and enforced dependency. It contributes to the development of mutual trust, openness of communication, cooperation and acceptance of responsibility.

STRATEGIES FOR HEALTH TEACHING

Step 3.   *Selecting appropriate educational strategies for goal attainment*

Ask yourself what strategies will work best to meet the educational objective for your patient. What resources are available, how much time do you and the learner have? What are the constraints and limitations of the strategy? How much effort do you predict will be needed to result in a successful performance? Is there a better way of achieving the same effect? Here are some strategies used for effective health teaching.

1. Write *all* instructions down clearly and concisely. Medication instructions should include trade and generic names, dosage, action, side effects and administration times. Include your name, the physician and a phone number for the client to call if necessary. Identify the appropriate actions and side effects.
2. Review instructions with the patient and significant family members. Paste the pill onto the instruction sheet.
3. Rehearse a performance with the learner and a significant other, for example, pulse taking, BP taking.
4. Tailor medication schedules with other home routines, for example, mealtimes.
5. Use sustained action prepared medications to reduce frequency of medication administration: once daily doses rather than bid, qid.
6. For symptom review, record of weight loss, or cigarette smoking pattern reduction have the learner keep a diary. This log gives the learner insight into his behavior and acts as a teaching tool by changing behavior.
7. Make weekly phone calls as a reminder about clinic appointments, to review a therapy or to allow for questions. Post cards as a reminder of clinic visits.
8. Use tailored educational tools according to a patient's reading level.
9. Make calendars for medication schedules or clinic appointments.
10. Provide daily medication schedules.
11. Support peer visits, for example, Reach for Recovery, Ostomy Association and laryngectomy groups.
12. Role play with the learner and/or significant other.
13. Use pill dispensers (similar to birth control pill dispenser).
14. Have peer group therapy sessions.
15. Use public health nursing for consultation to evaluate and reinforce the discharge plan.

Review the following cases, which depict the first three steps of the process presented thus far.

Case Presentation 1:

Problem: Discharge medications—prevention of noncompliance

Subjective Data: "I've had a pretty bad heart attack." "I don't know what heart medications I'm supposed to take when I go home." "I guess I have got to take heart pills to prevent another one of those heart attacks." "I'll do anything the doctor asks me to do." "I don't want to come back in here." "You know I stopped taking the pills my doctor gave me last year for my pressure because I didn't think I needed to take them all the time." "My wife is a nurse and she can help me with any questions I may have." "What do I have to do when I go home?" "What pills will I have to take?" "In order to get back to my law firm I need to know what I'm supposed to do."

Objective Data: The patient has an uncomplicated MI. Patient's health insurance will pay for all his cardiac medications. The CCU/PCU nurses do stress the need for medication compliance, are providing transportation for bimonthly clinic appointments, are reviewing the medication meal schedule, assisting him with pulse taking and other identified activities on a daily basis. Patient can read and graduated from high school.

Assessment: Patient and family need information about the medications the patient will be taking at home and appropriate decision making with which they may be confronted.

Plan: 1. History of patient's administration of medication
    A. Medications taken and medications prescribed
    B. Identification, by name preferably
    C. Knowledge of rationale
    D. Administration times and prescribed times
    E. Knowledge of side effects, warning signs
    F. Evaluation of adherence
  2. Core content
    A. Action and rationale
    B. Administration times
    C. Warning signs, side effects
    D. Appropriate decision making
  3. Method of teaching
    A. One-to-one instruction
    B. Recall evaluated
    C. Written instructions and daily schedule
    D. Significant other instructed
    E. Reinforcement with rehearsal
    F. Role play with side effects and possible situations patients will be faced with

Plan Objectives:
  Learning objectives:
1. The patient and family will be able to identify the rationale for the prescribed medications, stating the action of the medication and its effect on the patient's signs and symptoms generated by his heart attack.
2. The patient and family will be able to identify by name his prescribed medications, their administration times, corresponding with meals using the alarm clock.
3. The patient will be able to process his own complaints associated with his discharge medications, identifying warning signs and side effects of discharge medications, appropriate patient actions, and needs for available feedback by phoning physician, CCU, clinic nurse, or going to the emergency room.

4. The patient will be able to identify why it is important to adhere to the prescribed medication until otherwise stated, identifying the cost benefit of administering the medications.

Case Presentation 2:

Problem: Cigarette smoking. Following admission to the hospital the MI patient continues to smoke.

Subjective Data: This is the first admission for this 38-year-old married construction worker following the onset of crushing chest pain, sweating and nausea after a 12-hour delay on the job before seeking medical care. Risk factors include smoking and high blood pressure. No prior history of cardiac disease. The patient stated that he has had a "heart attack." "I don't know how bad it is." "I cannot see how quitting smoking can reduce my chances of a heart attack." "Even if I wanted to, I wouldn't know how to quit." "I've tried several times before." "I've never felt better, like a million dollars." "I have trouble with my pressure but can't stay on that diet that they gave me." "My wife smokes and if I do try to quit it would be hard to because I would be tempted by the smell of smoke in the house." "My doctor said I really should quit if I wanted to live longer." "Gee, I don't even know how many cigarettes I do smoke—I guess about two to three packs, usually after meals."

Objective Data: Smokes 2 ppd on hospital ward; uncomplicated transmural MI; no further chest pain since admission. Has health insurance. CCU/PCU nurses and primary physician stress the need to quit smoking. However, primary physician and primary nurse both smoke. Wife quit smoking two days ago. Patient's coworkers smoke on the job. Patient obtains cigarettes from visitors.

Assessment: Unaware of risk of smoking with MI. Patient needs assistance with smoking reduction plan.

Plan: 1. Assessment of patient's pattern of cigarette smoking during a 24-hour period, including time, number, circumstance, and rating of how one felt
2. Motivating factor introduced
3. Introduction of models of new behavior
4. Guided practice
5. Artificial reinforcement
6. Maintenance without reinforcement

Plan Objectives:

Learning objectives:
1. The patient will be able to identify the number of cigarettes smoked during a 24-hour period, including the frequency and circumstance, and rate from 1 to 4 how he felt.
2. The patient will identify the rationale for decreased smoking by identifying the risk of smoking and CAD, the severity of his condition, and the cost benefit of quitting smoking.
3. The patient will be able to identify the steps of the plan for new model behavior.
4. The patient will be able to identify and engage in the following activities to replace the need for a cigarette:
   A. reading, handcrafts, drinking beverages, brushing teeth, chewing gum.
   B. discuss conflict with spouse or significant other.
   C. have weekly discussion with CCU-PCU cardiac patients informing them of the need to quit smoking.

5. The patient will identify services available for guided practice:
   A. group sessions at cardiac clinic.
   B. cardiac clinic nurse—weekly appointments and phone calls.
   C. written discharge instructions.
   D. 24-hour available CCU phone service.
6. The patient will identify available artificial reinforcement:
   A. buying himself a gift weekly with the money saved by quitting smoking.
   B. spouse and family support.
   C. weekly group support—patient peer group.
   D. cardiac clinic nurse-physician support—bimonthly clinic appointments.

Step 4.   Evaluation of educational goal attainment and rediagnosis of educational needs

At this time it is necessary to evaluate your effectiveness as the educator, determining what has been learned and what the future educational needs of the learner and his family are. There are five steps that will enable you to evaluate your educational objectives.

Pearl (13) Evaluation of Health Teaching

1. *Effort.* This is the quantity of activity put forth by the teacher to educate the learner and effect compliance. You can determine this by documenting the frequency and duration of time spent by the nurse teaching the learner, as well as the cost of materials used. Are the learner's limitations too great to overcome? Can you predict success with the performance?

2. *Performance.* The result of the effort is defined as the performance. When reviewing your teaching, ask yourself, "How much was done?" and "What remains to be done?" (i.e., was it more effective to use the film or the one-to-one instruction in meeting the objective?) Will compliance be attained?

3. *Adequacy.* Was enough time spent on certain aspects of the content? Was there a need for reinforcement by weekly phone calls or more frequent clinic visits?

4. *Efficiency.* Is there a better way of achieving the same effect? Can group teaching give you the same outcome as one-to-one instruction, or was the film just as effective as a review of a teaching booklet by the learner and teacher?

5. *Process.* Why did the educational strategy work one way for one learner and not for another? What are the attributes of your strategy? What type of patient does it *not* work for? Who does it work for? What is the context of the situation in which it worked? What can be altered in the process to effect change and achieve the objective?

In the beginning of this chapter it was stressed that the major emphasis was on the *process* of health teaching. Now from familiarizing yourself with some of the salient points of the *process* which is so intimately involved in health teaching, adapt the steps involved in meeting the demands of the individual situations as you encounter them in your nursing role.

It is the fond hope of this author that these Pearls will serve as a guide in enabling you to reduce patient morbidity through your health educational efforts as an essential part of nursing care.

Pearl (14) Patient Teaching Worksheet

When you have a patient who may need teaching, such as the cardiac or ostomy patient, the newly diagnosed or the diabetic patient who has been readmitted, do you often find you are at a loss in deciding what must be taught, when and by whom?

To save time, avoid unnecessary repetition, reinforce specific aspects, and provide more effective communication in patient teaching among your staff, develop and use a "patient teaching worksheet." This can be placed in front of the patient's chart on a clipboard to hold these worksheets.

Also, the patient teaching worksheet can be placed on Kardex cards and held in the Kardex. Such a sheet also serves to establish evaluation criteria of the teaching and as a tool for the initial assessment of the patient's teaching needs, in order to establish priority of areas to be emphasized and those which need not be covered at all (see the chart below).

PATIENT TEACHING WORKSHEET FOR THE OSTOMY PATIENT	DATE	STAFF'S INITIALS	REMARKS
1. Stoma bag changed			
a. Patient observed			
b. Specific concerns of patient needing to continue to express			
c. Type bag			
d. Skin condition			
2. View film of ostomy care			
a. Understands anatomy			
b. Family watched film			
3. Colostomy booklet and packet			
4. Desire to have visitor from ostomy association			
5. Patient can:			
a. Remove stoma bag			
b. Cleanse skin			
c. Reapply bag			
d. Apply stoma belt, etc.			

PEARLS FOR TEACHING PATIENTS WITH PVD

Pearl (15) Adhere to Principles

The major principles which must be considered in teaching patients with peripheral vascular disease (PVD) are:
1. Prevent ischemia or further circulatory impairment caused by constricting gadgets and poor positioning.
2. Prevent infection in the extremities due to poor foot hygiene, irritating agents, or physical irritants.
3. Prevent emboli—the clot can be dislodged with improper care.
4. Decrease pain without impeding circulation and/or producing drug dependence.

Pearl (16) Specific Behaviors

Some specific points which should be emphasized that adhere to the principles include the following:

1. Wear white, cotton socks.
2. Use pumice stone to soften calluses and roughened skin on heels.
3. Dry feet thoroughly (wiping between each toe) and push the cuticles back, *gently.*
4. Use of oil (i.e., baby oil, keri oil, etc.) in the water to soak feet is also helpful.
5. *No* cutting of the nails with improper equipment (*no pocket knives* as some men often use), and never cut them too short. (Nails should be trimmed with nail clippers straight across not at angles.)
6. *Do not massage the legs*—this can dislodge the clot.
7. *Do not use heating pad, hot water bottle or light cradles on the extremities.* (This increases the metabolism in an already impaired circulatory area producing further ischemia and injury.)
8. Use lotion or skin cream to help relieve dryness.
9. Do not attempt to self-treat an injury or sore. Clean with antiseptic agent and consult physician.
10. Buy shoes which do not rub or cause physical irritation to the feet. It is best to alternate wearing a different pair of shoes every day. The pair not worn should be opened for airing.
11. Do not use constricting girdles, garters, belts or knee hose, which will further impair circulation.
12. Observe for any changes in circulation in the legs, such as coolness, increased pain, pain which awakens the patient from sleep, pain occurring on shorter periods of walking or standing, low back pain, or color changes.
13. Use a bath thermometer to check temperature of the water.

INSTRUCTIONAL SITUATIONS
Pearl (17) Simple Written Instructions for Routines

For those routines which are commonly performed on your specific unit, provide simple written instructions to facilitate the staff in their teaching. Refer to the notice regarding "24-hour Urine Collection."

24-HOUR URINE COLLECTION

Dear Patient,

You have been scheduled for a 24-hour urine collection test for

_____

by your physician. Please be sure to follow the instructions explained below.

1. Urinate to empty your bladder and flush the toilet to discard this urine. Write the exact time you urinated (to the minute) in the spaces provided.

Date _____ Time _____.

2. During the next 24-hours save ALL of your urine for the 24-hour collection test. Preservatives are added if needed.

To do this, urinate into the container in the bathroom (note Figure 11-4). Pour it directly into the collection bottle which may be kept on ice (note Figure 11-5).

3.   The last time you urinate, pour it into the collection bottle, this should be the next day, 24-hours after you began the test, written in #1 above.

4.   The urine collection bottle is kept in the bathroom for your convenience and to protect it from heat and sunlight. The nurse will send the collection bottle to the lab at the end of the test.

5.   If you should leave the unit for tests, x-rays, or other procedures during the collection period, please notify the nurse. She can give you a urine specimen bottle in case you need to urinate while you are off the unit.

If you need assistance or have any questions, please be sure to ask. If by accident any urine is lost, please be sure to notify the nurse immediately.
Thank you!
Ambulatory Unit Nursing Staff
Written by: Ada Cowwins, L.P.N., 1976; Shands Teaching Hospital

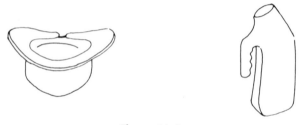

Figure 11-4

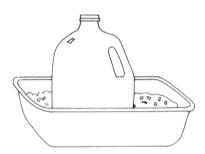

Figure 11-5

Pearl (18) Those Floating Contacts

A scratched cornea, infection and even impaired vision are some of the complications which can occur with the inadequate care of the patient who wears contact lenses.

Consider these suggestions in assuring safe care of the patient with contact lenses:

1.   Too often the patient, on removing a contact lens which has slipped off the cornea or who had an irritant, such as dust in his eye, moistens the lens with his *saliva*

and replaces it. This practice should be discouraged due to the potential for infection. He should moisten the lens with a sterile ophthalmic solution. This can be carried in his lens case and placed in the pocket or purse.

2.   When corneal lenses are removed, place them in a lens case or in separate containers with water or sterile ophthalmic solution. Be certain to place the correct lens in the correct side (left or right) of the case or in similarly labeled containers.

3.   When you are removing the contact lens from the patient's eye, be careful to prevent injury to the eye.

Pearl (19) Apply "Specs" Safely

The patient should be taught to take hold of each ear piece with one hand and put the glasses over the ears. It is essential that a patient *does not* hold the glasses near the frames and attempt to slide them on, along the side of the face. Why? The frame edges might strike him in the eye.

USE OF A MODEL HOSPITAL
Pearl (20) A Model Hospital—Where the Doll Goes to Surgery

A model hospital was designed by Ms. Mary Lynn, R.N., to help orient children awaiting surgery to the operating and recovery rooms.

While a tour would help them become familiar with the unknown areas, the hospital model would have additional advantages. Basic premises of the model:

1.   It should be less stressful than a tour of the actual operating room and recovery room. Sensory overload would be less likely.
2.   The child would receive about the same information as a tour.
3.   It would be a play activity in which the child would be in control of the situation as he pushes the doll on its stretcher through the model hospital.
4.   There would be more time and occasions to reflect and to push the doll through the model hospital. This should promote questions and comments by the child.

REFERENCES

Becker, M. H. and Maiman, L. A. "Socio-Behavioral Determinants of Compliance with Health and Medical Care Recommendations." *Medical Care* 13:10-24, 1975.

Mager, Robert F. *Preparing Instructional Objectives.* Palo Alto, Calif.: Fearon Pubs., 1962.

Sackett, David L. and Haynes, R. Brian. *Compliance with Therapeutic Regimes.* Baltimore, Md.: Johns Hopkins University Press, 1976.

Unpublished works:

Fass, Marion. "Educational Diagnosis." Lecture presented at the Workshop on "Patient Education" February, 1977, in Worcester, Mass.

Zapka, Jane. "Evaluation." Lecture presented at the Workshop on "Patient Education" February, 1977, in Worcester, Mass.